The 10-Minute Physical Exam

recognizing medical syndromes

Clifford Chan-Yan MBChB, FRCPC

Eldon Underhill Illustrator

For information, contact:
Clifford Chan-Yan
email cliffchanyan@telus.net
phone 604-209-0279

Notice: This book contains information obtained from authentic and highly regarded sources. While reasonable efforts have been made to publish reliable information, neither the authors nor the publisher can accept any legal responsibility or liability for any errors or omissions that may be made. The publishers wish to make clear that any views or opinions expressed in this book by individual editors, authors, or contributors are personal to them and do not necessarily reflect the views/opinions of the publishers. The information or guidance contained in this book is intended for use by medical, scientific, or health care professionals and is provided strictly as a supplement to medical or other professionals' own judgment and their knowledge of a patient's medical history. If any copyright material has not been acknowledged, we apologize; please write and let us know so that we may rectify it in any future reprint.

ISBN (paperback) 978-1-7774503-1-1
ISBN (electronic) 978-1-7774503-0-4

Cover design and illustrations by Eldon Underhill
Page design and layout by Vancouver Desktop Publishing Centre

Printed in the United States by IngramSpark

Remembering Angus Ian Rae, colleague, friend, Master Clinician

In the fields of observation chance favors only the prepared mind

—Louis Pasteur

Contents

PART ONE: The 10-Minute Physical Exam

CARDIOLOGY 37

ENDOCRINOLOGY 51

GASTROENTEROLOGY 65

HEMATOLOGY / ONCOLOGY 77

INFECTIOUS DISEASE 91

Foreword

There has been an expanding body of manuals over the decades that provide instruction on physical examination, each describing the detailed maneuvers that may be performed with each body system. Why, then, are the physical exam skills of clinicians continuing to decline? It appears to be due, in large part, to a downward spiral of decreasing confidence in physical examinations and increasing dependence on technological tests for diagnosis. How may clinicians' confidence and competence in physical examination be restored? More of the same is not working. Although technological testing is becoming increasingly sophisticated, physical examination can often detect important signs that suggest or make a diagnosis or that direct rational investigations and appropriate referrals. Importantly, it nurtures the special healing and reassuring relationship between patient and physician that is rewarding to both.

A potential problem of current training is that medical students may be graduating with physical examination skills that are underdeveloped, and without evidence that their abilities might improve after entering clinical practice. They are introduced to physical examination early during training and are expected to observe for lists of signs that are often out of context for the clinical situations they encounter. Ongoing review and assessment of their skills are typically lacking during the remaining years of training, when competence and confidence in performing physical examinations could develop in the context of clinical experience. Remarkably, many trainees state that they have not observed a clinician demonstrating a general examination and do not know what is realistic and acceptable. As a result, physical examination becomes disorganized and superficial. It is necessary for medical programs to address this notable deficiency. This will require organization, resources, and recruitment of clinicians committed to physical examination.

In *The 10-Minute Physical Exam*, Dr. Chan-Yan maintains that competent physical examination need not entail all the comprehensive maneuvers specific to each body system. Rather, it should be an efficient screen of the whole body, performed consistently, with permission to abbreviate and modify maneuvers but to also supplement them with greater detail when warranted. He notes that the skilled surgeon determines the organization of the surgical tray before proceeding to perform an operation with predetermined sequence and effort-sparing efficiency. So too with physical examination—preparation, orderly sequence, consistency, and relaxed efficiency are necessary. The examination is choreographed in 4 mini-exams, each to be practiced and perfected before combining them into a single fluid routine, lessening the likelihood of missing important diagnostic clues.

A novel addition to the manual is the inclusion of 51 medical syndromes, each with a list of clinical signs and matching annotated patient figures, illustrated by Underhill. Knowing and recognizing the clinical signs of medical conditions are essential attributes of the diagnostician. Readers are encouraged to review these syndromes and to add their own on the extra blank pages.

The 10-Minute Physical Exam provides a fresh approach to conducting physical exams that is well presented and attractively illustrated.

Julio S. G. Montaner, OC, OBC, MD, DSc (hon), FRCPC, FCCP, FACP, FRSC
Killam Professor, Division of Infectious Diseases, Faculty of Medicine,
  University of British Columbia
Executive Director and Physician-in-Chief, BC Centre for Excellence
  in HIV/AIDS
Head, HIV/AIDS Program, St. Paul's Hospital, Providence Health Care
UBC and St. Paul's Foundation Chair in AIDS Research

Introduction

"You can observe a lot by just watching."

—Yogi Berra

Why a Routine and Why a Manual?

A screening physical examination can easily be completed in 10 minutes or less. All it takes is an efficient routine and a modicum of practice.

This manual provides guidance on a series of 4 mini-exams that can be choreographed into a seamless routine to assess key body parts and systems with minimal effort and repetition. Once the routine becomes fluid, and with baseline experience developed through practice, you will be able to identify clinical signs that might suggest a diagnosis, warrant greater detail to a particular body system, or direct specific laboratory investigations.

This manual comprises 2 parts:

- **Part One** introduces the 4 mini-exams and the routine that underlies *The 10-Minute Physical Exam*. Each mini-exam is presented in terms of the patient's physical position during the exam, targeted body areas, examination of patient movements and reflexes, and flow from one assessment to the next.

- **Part Two** is a compendium of illustrated medical syndromes with associated clinical signs that may be observed during the physical exam. Awareness and recognition of the clinical signs of medical syndromes are the cornerstones of effective diagnosis.

What is not in this manual:

- Instruction is not provided on the standard maneuvers that must be learned to perform a physical examination, but which are covered in many available books. (The exception is testing of the tendon reflexes, which is included in the manual as it is often performed awkwardly and ineffectively.)

The emphasis here is on the development of a repeatable and efficient exam sequence. Mastery of the 10-minute physical exam routine then allows you to refine detailed exam maneuvers that can be incorporated, as necessary, into the exam sequence.

Physical Examination: A Perspective

Instruction on conducting a physical examination typically occurs early during medical school training, when our clinical knowledge and experience are limited. Often, we are taught how to examine different body systems at different times and by different tutors but are not shown how to integrate this into an overall screening exam. Remarkably, students and residents often state that they have not observed a clinician performing a screening physical exam. Even as we acquire knowledge and experience through later years of training, there is no formal review or evaluation of our physical exam skills. And with no formal instruction or learning, there follows a lack of practice of the skills that are most useful in clinical diagnosis.

We are taught to perform comprehensive physical examinations, which include consciously seeking or excluding lists of physical signs that are out of context for the clinical situation. When physical exams are not problem focused, we develop hesitant and lasting random habits.

Unfortunately, there is no evidence that physical exam skills naturally improve in the years after graduation—that is, without additional training and consolidation of knowledge. As with any skill, physical exam skills need to be taught, learned, practiced, and perfected. With patient rounds increasingly being conducted in hallways, at computer terminals, and in conference rooms, there is little to no time set aside for the bedside review of clinical signs. And without confidence in our ability to adequately perform physical exams, we are more likely to rely on special tests rather than the physical signs that could dictate diagnosis and management.

It is telling that, a hundred years ago, a clinician could detect all the signs of pericardial effusion, the diagnosis of which may challenge a modern-day physician without access to an echocardiogram.

What, then, is the solution? Reaffirmation among clinicians and educators of the value of the physical exam in diagnosis, treatment, and management is an important step. This requires competent and committed clinicians to provide the initial training, to assess students' skills, and to mentor them through early and later stages of their career. Physical exam skills should be reviewed and assessed periodically throughout training and should be honed and maintained throughout one's later clinical practice.

The other aspect of the solution is to follow a consistent routine that efficiently screens all body systems while allowing for more detailed evaluation of a system when clinically indicated. By screening the whole body, easily detectable clinical signs that are possibly diagnostic are less likely to be missed.

Telemedicine and the Physical Exam

Telemedicine evolved slowly over several decades until the COVID-19 pandemic caused an explosion of interest in developing digital health strategies.

While traditional medical care is provided almost exclusively via in-person interactions between patients and health care professionals, telemedicine involves remote patient care through the use of telecommunications technologies. Access to the internet and advances in digital technology now commonly support these remote interactions, ranging from phone calls, to digital communications, to real-time online visits with video capabilities, and even to procedures conducted through remotely controlled equipment.

Telemedicine provides a number of advantages over traditional medicine: broader availability of health care access for remote and rural communities, increased efficiency of health care delivery in cases where care is independent of physical evaluations, ease of chronic disease monitoring and management, and convenience in terms of reduced travel time and cost.

There is one key drawback, however, in that effective physical exams are not possible with telemedicine. As such, and given the importance of physical exam in patient evaluation and diagnosis, telemedicine and in-person health care will continue to be complementary. In-person health care also provides an avenue for the supportive healing and reassurance that patients often receive from being examined physically (by touch), not just verbally (by voice) or visually by limited observations (by sight and through remote systems).

With fewer in-person office visits come fewer opportunities for clinicians to develop their physical examination skills. And so, manuals such as this, which support the efficient examination of key body parts and systems, and which consolidate various clinical signs into specific medical diagnoses, are a critical piece of the collective knowledge bank of proficient clinicians.

An Illustrative Clinical Case

There are frequent instances when medical diagnoses are made by conducting batteries of special tests but when the patients are retroactively visited at the bedside, it becomes evident that diagnostic clues could have been detected with a basic screening physical exam.

In many cases, physical exams are not performed during early attempts at diagnosis or they are performed in a cursory manner or are unstructured. Potential diagnostic "clues" detected at the bedside can direct more focused body system examinations and result in judiciously selected special tests.

Consider the following clinical case.

A 19-year-old, Asian female was referred for symptoms of malaise and intermittent low-grade fever. Physical examination was reported by 2 clinicians as unremarkable. Laboratory tests revealed mild microcytic anemia, weakly positive antinuclear antibody, mild polyclonal gammaglobulinemia, elevated C-reactive protein, and negative blood cultures. Chest X-ray and abdominal ultrasound were reported normal.

At the referred visit, the patient was afebrile with mild conjunctival pallor. A physical exam was initiated, starting with the upper extremities and including simultaneous bilateral palpation of the radial pulses. This revealed a faint pulse on the left side, with a left brachial systolic blood pressure of 50 mmHg and a right brachial pressure of 98/50 mmHg. Auscultation revealed a bruit over the right carotid artery, which was palpably rigid. The left carotid artery pulsation was diminished, with a systolic bruit. The remainder of the examination was unremarkable.

At this stage of the examination, within less than 5 minutes, the most likely diagnosis was Takayasu's arteritis.

Even if a clinician was not familiar with Takayasu's arteritis, the striking findings of asymmetric radial pulses and blood pressures along with carotid bruits would immediately direct investigation at the arterial system. Instead of laboratory tests, it was a habitually routine, efficient physical exam that ensured the body systems were appropriately screened. In this case, Takayasu's arteritis was confirmed by MR angiography and appropriate treatment was prescribed. The striking diagnostic signs had been hiding in plain sight.

Why might important detectable clinical signs be missed, or why might the physical exam be omitted?

A variety of reasons include lack of clinician competence or confidence, a predetermined expectation of not detecting anything significant, or the belief that physical exam is inherently unreliable. Superficial examination of the patient and randomness from one exam to the next ensue. However, the skilled surgeon plans ahead, determines organization of the surgical tray, and proceeds in an efficient and expeditious manner. Similarly, the key to an efficient physical exam is to perform it with an established efficient and orderly routine and with mind wide open.

PART ONE

The 10-Minute Physical Exam

"Learn to see, learn to hear, learn to feel, learn to smell, and know that by practice alone you can become expert."
—*Sir William Osler*

Position 1

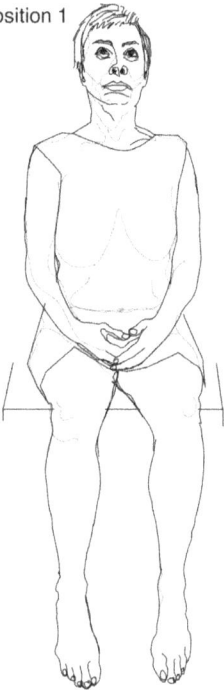

Position 2

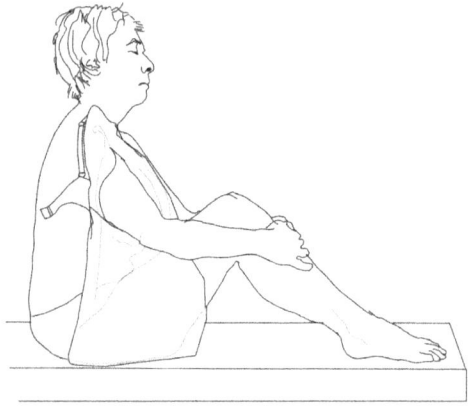

Position 3

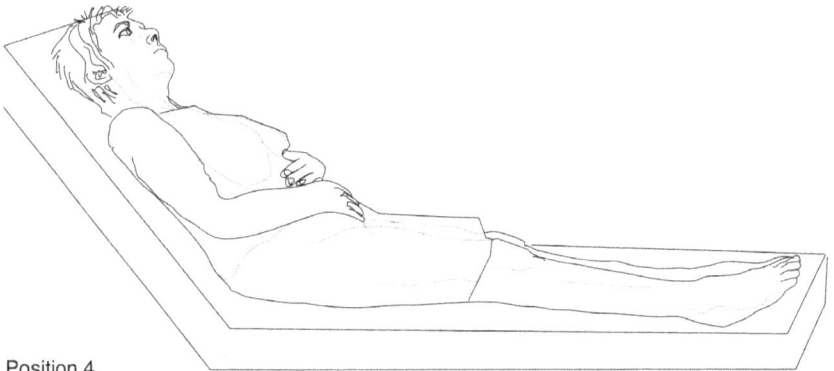

Position 4

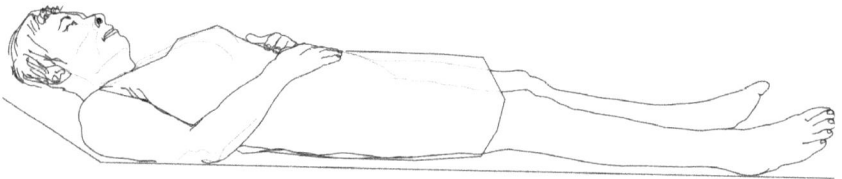

The 4 mini-exam positions

The 10-Minute Physical Exam

A meaningful and effective screening physical exam can be accomplished in less than 10 minutes. The key to this is an efficient routine that screens the whole body, minimizes physical effort and repetition, and is tailored to individual clinician preferences and specific clinical scenarios. In terms of the routine, this requires consistency in the sequence of actions and in their repeated application—both of which take practice.

The Exam

The overall physical exam consists of 4 mini-exams, each corresponding to a different physical position that the patient adopts. Ultimately, the mini-exams are integrated into a rapid, seamless routine that provides an assessment of the whole body.

For each mini-exam, you should practice the evaluations and commit the sequence to memory, with a focus on identifying any findings that appear abnormal or restricted.

Mini-Exam	Patient Position on Examination Table	Target Body Areas
1	Seated, with legs hanging over edge of table	Upper extremities, head, neck, including visual fields
2	Seated, with legs extended along length of table	Spine, posterior chest
3	Semi-reclined at about 40 degrees	Jugular veins, anterior chest, heart
4	Lying supine	Abdomen, lower extremities

The "how to" for each of these mini-exams is presented in the following sections.

The instruction for each mini-exam focuses on (i) the appropriate use of the exam gown and drape, (ii) the actions and/or movements that the patient is asked to follow along with the actions and observations performed by the clinician, (iii) the techniques for testing reflexes (where applicable), and (iv) the performance of the mini-exam while incorporating the aforementioned. Importantly, attention is drawn to the patient's actions and movements and not just to the static examination positions.

Routine Takes Practice

The approach presented in this guide leads to an effective and efficient physical exam that is appropriate for screening purposes. The focus is on learning an examination sequence (routine) that can be followed easily and with increasing fluidity. As the routine becomes second nature, you will become more observant of abnormal or unexpected clinical signs in the patients you are examining. These signs serve to direct a more focused body part or body system examination or may suggest a specific diagnosis.

Building the routine takes practice: practice in instructing the patient's actions and movements, practice in effortlessly performing the reflex tests (e.g., on first try), practice in following the sequence of events (i.e., following the script), and practice in pulling the mini-exams together and integrating the findings. It is also equally important to practice the exam on a variety of patients (different sex, age, build, etc.), as well as in different settings such as clinics and hospital wards.

The exam routine is flexible and adaptable to different scenarios—while it includes several techniques that have been modified for screening purposes, these can easily be supplemented by standard examination maneuvers as appropriate.

Exam Gown

Use of the exam gown and drape sheet deserves special attention. For an exam to be effective, it is often necessary to obtain full but discrete exposure of the body area in question while respecting patient modesty and privacy. Best practice involves the following:

- Offering a gown to all patients (regardless of sex, age, etc.)
- Requesting the patient to undress down to their underwear and to put the gown on open to the back and loosely tied (if applicable, requesting that undergarments with straps be loosened and/or clasps undone)
- Providing a drape across the pelvis and upper legs

In each case, exposure should be limited to the body part being examined. Specific considerations for gown use and drapery are provided for each mini-exam.

Mini-Exam 1

Patient Position   Seated, with legs hanging over edge of examination table

Target Body Areas   Upper extremities
Head
Neck
Visual fields

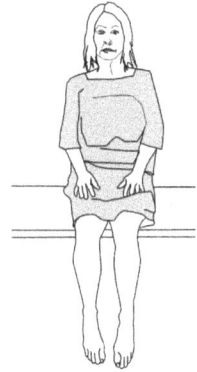

This mini-exam involves a series of actions and movements by the patient and an evaluation of upper extremity tendon reflexes by the clinician. A quick screen of visual fields is included in this mini-exam.

Position and Exam Gown

For Mini-Exam 1, the patient is seated upright on the table with their legs hanging down, with the exam gown open at the back and loosely tied, and with a drape across their upper legs.

Actions and Movements (by Patient)

1. Patient places hands behind head, followed by hands behind back.

> **Quick screen for:**
> - hands behind head: arm abduction, elbow flexion, shoulder external rotation
> - hands behind back: arm adduction, elbow flexion, shoulder internal rotation

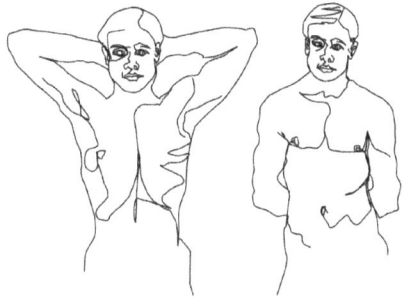

2. Patient crosses forearms and firmly hooks index and middle fingers together with your index and middle fingers (patient's right hand with your right, and left hand with your left hand). Against resistance, patient attempts to pull hands apart and extend arms.

> **Quick screen for:**
> - hand grip, arm strength

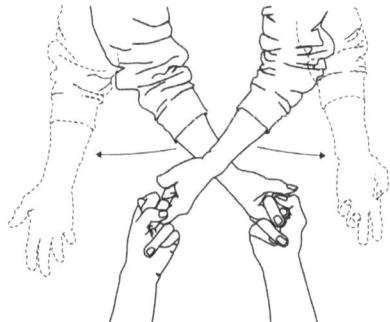

3. Patient performs the finger-nose test, followed by rapid pronation-supination of hands.

Quick screen for:
- cerebellar coordination

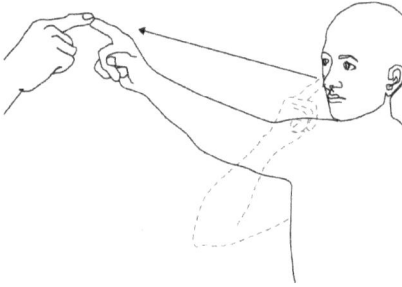

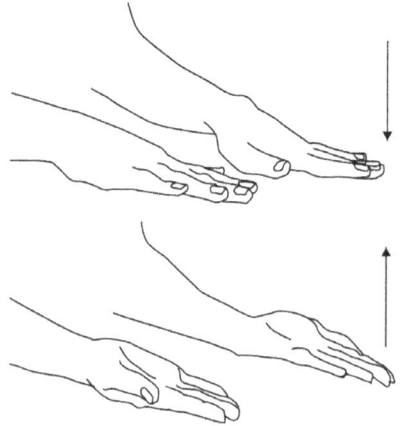

4. Patient looks down and up, then turns head to one side and then the other side.

Quick screen for:
- neck flexion and extension, neck rotation

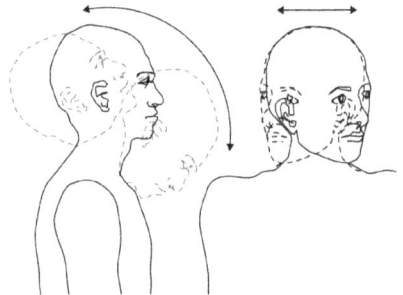

Tendon Reflex Tests (by Clinician)

Ensure that the patient's arm is relaxed.

1. Brachioradialis (supinator) reflex

In Position 1, the patient's hands will naturally be resting on their upper thighs. Place your first two fingers across the lower end of the patient's radius, just above the styloid. Firmly tap your fingers with the reflex hammer as your fingers are held against the tendon.

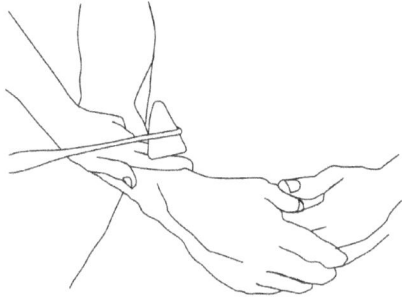

2. Biceps reflex

The patient's elbows will be slightly flexed, with hands resting on their upper thighs. Clasp the patient's arm above the elbow, with your thumb across the tendon and fingers around the back of the arm. Firmly tap your thumb with the reflex hammer as your thumb is held against the tendon.

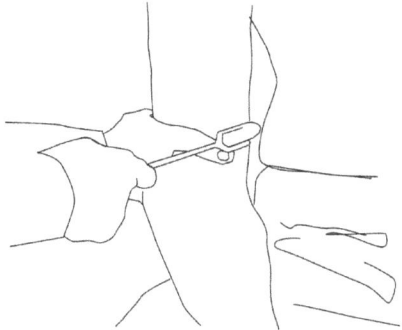

3. Triceps reflex

Lift and support the patient's elbow, allowing their forearm to rest along your forearm. Use the reflex hammer to tap the triceps tendon.

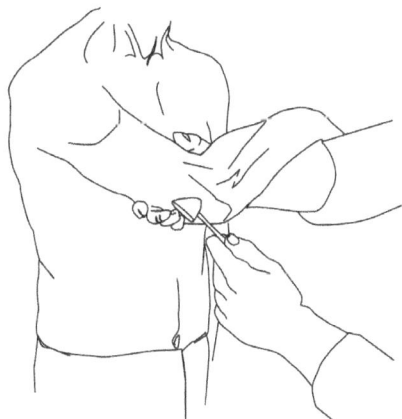

4. Quadriceps reflex (Option 1, also refer to Mini-Exam 4)

Position 1 is used to evaluate the upper extremities but is also convenient to test the lower extremity quadriceps reflex since the patient's legs are hanging over the side of the examination table.

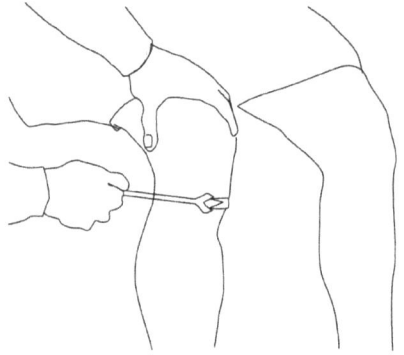

To test the quadriceps reflex at this stage of the exam, palpate for the tibial tuberosity, then use the reflex hammer to firmly tap the patellar tendon just above the tuberosity.

Visual Field Test (by Clinician)

You and the patient face each other, approximately 1 m apart and with eyes level. Have the patient cover one eye with their hand and look directly at you with the open eye (e.g., patient's left eye to your right eye). Close your eye that is opposite the patient's closed eye.

Hold up both your hands, equidistant from the patient, with your fingers at the periphery of the superior hemifield on each side of the eye's vertical midline. Move the fingers of one hand and ask the patient to indicate on which side there is movement. Repeat a couple of times, wiggling the fingers of one or both hands.

Repeat for the lower hemifield. Then repeat the test for the other eye.

Quick screen for:
- gross visual field defect

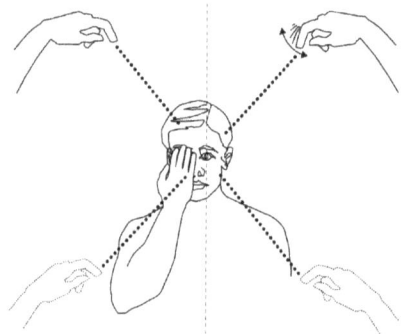

PERFORMING MINI-EXAM 1

Face the patient who is seated on the side of the examination table with their legs hanging down.

Upper extremities

- With fingers of both hands, simultaneously palpate both of the patient's radial pulses.

- Measure the blood pressure in each arm if this is a first visit, and periodically during subsequent physical exams.

- Instruct and demonstrate: "Place both hands behind your head, then behind your back."

- Instruct and demonstrate: "Cross your forearms and grip your first two fingers together with mine, your right hand with my right hand and your left hand with my left hand. Now, while I resist, try to uncross and straighten your arms."

- While still clasping hands, pull and push the patient's relaxed arms gently back and forth (checking muscle tone).

- Instruct and demonstrate: "Touch your nose with a finger then quickly touch my moving finger; repeat again, and again."

- Instruct and demonstrate: "Show me the palms of both hands, then quickly turn them over to show me the backs of both hands; quickly repeat palm up and palm down."

- Test for sense of touch by touching 3 or 4 spots on the hands and arms with a piece of cotton wool or tissue. Ask the patient if it feels normal.

- Test tendon reflexes:

  – Brachioradialis (supinator)

  – Biceps

  – Triceps

  – (Quadriceps option)

Head

- Instruct: "Turn your head to one side, then to the opposite side; now look to the sky and then down."

- Instruct: "Raise your eyebrows; now close your eyes; now show me your teeth" (CN VII); "stick out your tongue" (CN XII).

- Instruct: "Follow my finger with your eyes, up, down, to each side" (CN III, IV, VI, nystagmus).
- Instruct: "Repeat the number that I am going to whisper in each ear" (CN VIII).

Neck

- Auscultate the carotid arteries.
- Place your hands at the base of the patient's neck, with thumbs meeting close to or at the midline and fingers spread across the clavicles. Then perform the following:
  - Move your right thumb up to palpate the patient's left carotid artery; then do the same on the other side.
  - Move your right thumb down to smoothly palpate over the right lobe of the thyroid gland; repeat on the other side.
  - Palpate to check if the trachea is midline.
  - Palpate for supraclavicular and submandibular lymph nodes.

Visual fields

- Instruct: "Cover your right eye with your fingers and keep looking at my right eye. I will hold up fingers on both sides above your head. Tell me on which side my fingers are wiggling." Repeat for the lower hemifield, and for the other eye.
- Use an ophthalmoscope to scan the retina.

Mini-Exam 2

Patient Position   Seated, with legs extended along the length of the examination table

Target Body Areas   Spine
Posterior chest

This mini-exam involves 2 movements conducted by the patient to screen the spine and posterior chest. There are no tendon reflexes to be tested.

Position and Exam Gown

The patient is seated upright, with their legs along the examination table, with gown open and their back exposed.

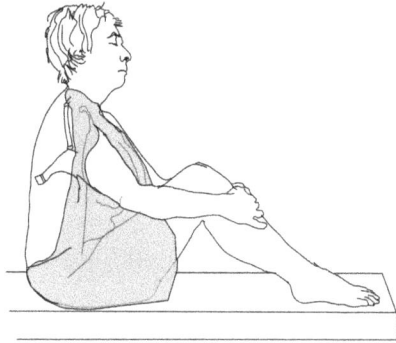

Actions and Movements (by Patient)

1. Patient rotates shoulders and trunk to one side, then to the other side.

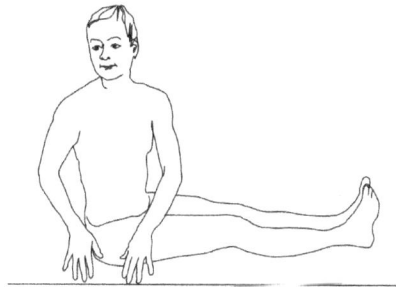

Quick screen for:
- rotation of the spine, with pelvis fixed on the examination table

2. Patient reaches forward to touch toes, with back arched.

Quick screen for:
- spine flexion, hip flexion

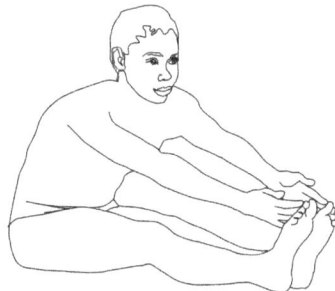

Tendon Reflex Tests (by Clinician)

None.

PERFORMING MINI-EXAM 2

Patient is seated in profile, with their legs along the length of the examination table. The patient's back is exposed through the gown that opens at the back.

Spine

- Inspect the back and run your fingers down the patient's spine to check for alignment and bony anomalies.
- Instruct: "Twist your shoulders and chest to one side, then the other side."
- Instruct: "Reach over to touch your toes; allow your back to arch."

Posterior chest

- Percuss and auscultate the posterior chest.

Mini-Exam 3

Patient Position   Semi-reclined (at approximately 40 degrees)

Target Body Areas   Jugular veins
Anterior chest
Heart

This mini-exam involves the clinician evaluating the jugular veins and anterior chest and heart while the patient is in a semi-reclined position. There are no active movements by the patient or tendon reflexes to be tested.

Position and Exam Gown

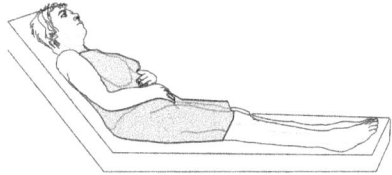

The patient is semi-reclined on the examination table. With consent, one side of the chest is briefly exposed for examination by removing one arm from the gown sleeve. If applicable, removal of the undergarment/bra straps is preferred to allow for unimpeded inspection and auscultation. Cover the chest and repeat on the opposite side.

Actions and Movements (by Patient)

None.

Tendon Reflex Tests (by Clinician)

None.

PERFORMING MINI-EXAM 3

The patient is semi-reclined, which provides visual access to the jugular veins. Placement of the gown is such that one side of the chest is exposed at a time to facilitate inspection and examination.

Jugular veins

- Assess the height of the jugular veins.

Anterior chest

- Inform and request: "I would like to examine the right side of your chest, listen to your lungs, and check your armpit for lymph nodes. If that is alright, please pull your arm out of the gown sleeve (and undergarment/ bra strap, if applicable)."

- On the right side:
  - Inspect the anterior chest.
  - Percuss and auscultate the right anterior and lateral chest.
  - Palpate the axilla for lymph glands.
- Have the patient reinsert their arm through the gown sleeve (and undergarment/bra strap, if applicable).
- Repeat procedure on the left side.

Heart

- Examine the heart while left side of chest remains exposed:
  - Locate and check the cardiac apical impulse.
  - Palpate the precordium.
  - Auscultate.
- Have the patient reinsert their arm through the gown sleeve (and undergarment/bra strap, if applicable.
- Carefully lower the head of the examination table, for the patient to lie supine in preparation for Mini-Exam 4.

Mini-Exam 4

Patient Position   Lying supine

Target Body Areas   Abdomen
                            Lower extremities

This mini-exam involves a series of actions and movements by the patient and an evaluation of the abdomen and lower extremity tendon reflexes by the clinician.

Position and Exam Gown

The patient is lying supine with gown pulled up to the costal margin and a drape placed across the pelvis and upper legs. The abdomen is exposed until abdomen screening is complete, and then the gown is lowered.

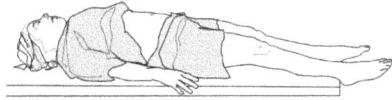

To expose the lower extremities, the patient remains supine and the drape is adjusted. The drape continues to cover the pelvis, with the lower section of the drape tucked between the upper thighs to expose the legs.

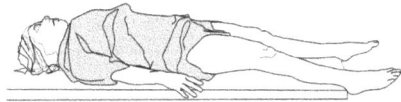

Actions and Movements (by Patient)

1. Patient pulls both knees to chest.

Quick screen for:
• hip flexion, knee flexion

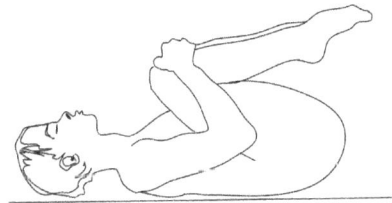

2. Patient draws one heel along the examination table toward the buttock, then drops the knee laterally toward the table. Repeat with the other leg.

Quick screen for:
• knee flexion, hip abduction, external rotation

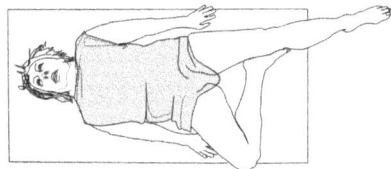

3. Patient places heel on the shin of the other leg and then slides the heel up and down, from the knee to the ankle. Repeat with the other heel and leg.

Quick screen for:
• cerebellar function

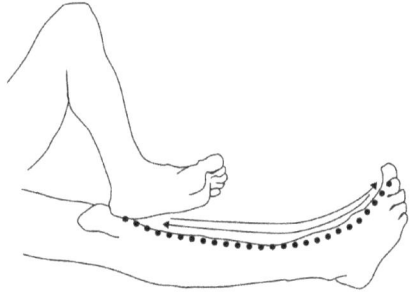

Tendon Reflex Tests (by Clinician)

1. Quadriceps reflex

   • Option 1 – It is often convenient to test the quadriceps reflex earlier in the overall routine as part of Mini-Exam 1 when the patient is seated with legs hanging over the side of the examination table. Palpate for the tibial tuberosity, then use the reflex hammer to firmly tap the patellar tendon just above the tuberosity (see Mini-Exam 1).

   • Option 2 – Patient is supine with both legs relaxed and knees slightly flexed. Support both legs with your hand and forearm and palpate the tibial tuberosity. With the reflex hammer, firmly tap the patellar tendon just above the tuberosity of each leg. If supporting both legs is awkward, raise one leg at a time.

   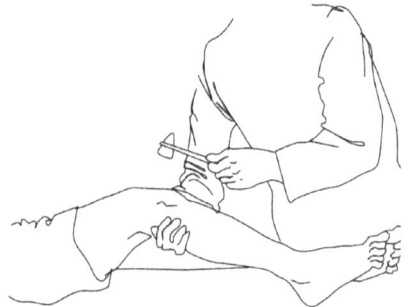

   • Option 3 – With patient's leg extended, place a finger across the cephalad edge of the patella, then use the reflex hammer to firmly tap on your finger caudally against the patella. Repeat with the other leg.

   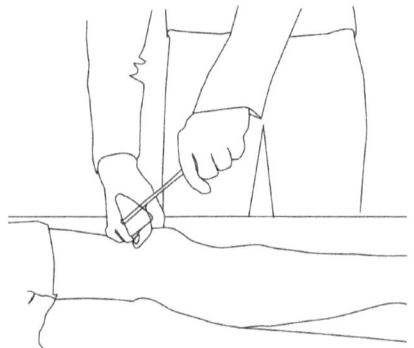

2. Achilles reflex

- Option 1 – With the patient's knee partially flexed and dropped toward the examination table, grasp the foot and slightly flex the ankle. With the reflex hammer, firmly tap the Achilles tendon.

- Option 2 – With patient's leg extended, grasp and hold the forefoot with your fingers across the plantar aspect. While holding the ankle in slight flexion, use the reflex hammer to firmly tap against your fingers, with your fingers held across the plantar aspect. This test is facilitated by holding the foot slightly everted (i.e., turned outward).

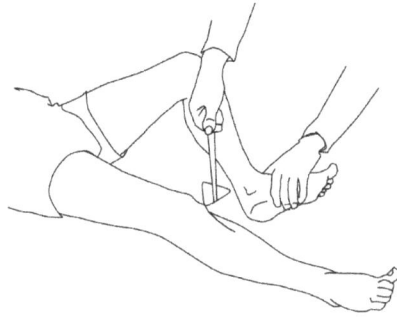

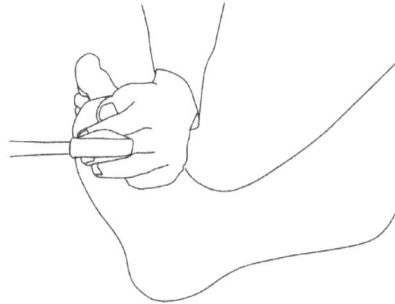

3. Plantar reflex

Use a stiff object, such as a key or edge of a thumb nail, to stroke the lateral aspect of the sole from the heel to the ball of the foot, curving medially across the ball.

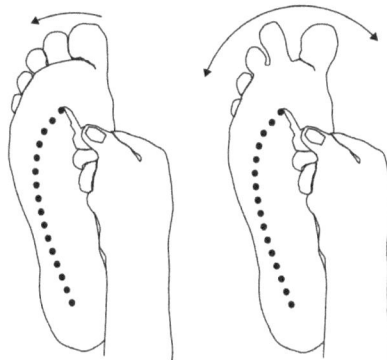

PERFORMING MINI-EXAM 4

The patient is lying supine with the gown adjusted to first expose the abdomen and then adjusted to expose the lower extremities while keeping the pelvis and groin draped.

Abdomen

- Expose the abdomen by raising the gown to the costal margin.

- Palpate lightly and continuously around the quadrants and along the midline. Repeat with deeper palpation to examine for masses.

- Palpate for the liver and spleen edges when you are at the upper quadrants. (It is not necessary to commence at the opposite lower quadrant if you are already able to define the liver and spleen edge.)

  - Attempt bimanual ballottement at each flank for the kidneys.

- Auscultate the abdomen. Move your stethoscope to each quadrant and to the midline to listen for bruits and bowel sounds.

- With the stethoscope still in your ears, inform the patient that you will auscultate over the femoral arteries. Auscultate over the femoral arteries, and palpate the inguinal areas for the femoral artery pulses and lymph nodes.

Lower extremities

- Cover the abdomen and expose the patient's legs with appropriate draping (e.g., tucking a drape section between the upper inner thighs).

- Instruct: "Bend your knees and pull them up to your chest with your hands."

- Instruct: "Pull your right heel toward your buttock, then drop your right knee toward the table. Repeat with your left leg."

- Instruct: "Straighten your legs and keep them relaxed as I move your knee, like this." Then quickly lift the knee up and off the table. Note if the heel drags along the table or lifts off the table (quick check for tone).

- Instruct: "While I hold each knee down, try to lift it off the table" (quick test for power).

- Instruct: "Place your right heel on your left shin and move it up and down between your knee and ankle. Repeat with the other heel" (quick check for cerebellar function).

- Test for sense of touch by touching 3 or 4 spots below the knee with a piece of cotton wool or tissue. Ask the patient if it feels normal.

- Palpate the posterior tibial and dorsalis pedal pulses.

- Test tendon reflexes:

  - Quadriceps

  - Achilles

  - Plantar

Putting It All Together:
The 10-Minute Physical Exam Sequence

Now it is time to integrate the 4 mini-exams into a single screening sequence. Practice the routine with the aim of minimizing repetition and effort and improving fluidity. Adapt specific actions, movements, and reflex tests depending on the setting (e.g., clinic, ward) and patient positioning or mobility. As the routine becomes familiar, shift your focus to observing for abnormal signs and restricted movements.

Start the exam after meeting the patient and taking an appropriate history. Perform the exam as follows:

- Note the patient's general appearance, demeanor, mobility, and gait.

- Explain that you will perform a general screening examination. The following can be included if predetermined with your patient or as a separate exam, if warranted:

  - Examination of the genitourinary and anorectal region

  - Female breast examination

- Provide an examination gown and request that the patient undress to their underwear and secure the gown loosely with the opening at the back.

- Begin with Mini-Exam 1 and work through Mini-Exams 2, 3, and 4 in sequence.

- At each step, note any abnormal signs, restricted movements, or abnormal reflexes.

- If something abnormal is detected, and if warranted, modify your examination for greater focus on the relevant body system.

PRACTICE POINT: Patients appreciate diligence and are reassured when they are physically examined.

While you are on clinical ward assignments, use the opportunity to practice the routine by requesting your patient's permission to perform a whole-body screening exam or a screening exam focused on a particular body system of interest. Repetition and application of the physical exam on a wide range of patient types helps you develop a broad reference set and enables you to be able to detect abnormalities and identify unexpected results. This information is critical in directing additional focused examinations and investigations.

The 10-Minute Physical Exam

Mini-Exam	Patient Position on Exam Table	Target Body Areas	Actions or Movements by Patient	Reflex Tests by Clinician	Other Elements of the Exam Routine
1	Seated, with legs hanging over edge of table	Upper extremities	• Hands behind head, and behind back • Crossed forearms, hooked fingers with examiner, undo against resistance • Finger-nose test, and hand pronation-supination	• Brachioradialis (supinator) • Biceps • Triceps • (Quadriceps option)	• Palpate radial pulses simultaneously • Measure blood pressure • Test for sense of touch
		Head and neck	• Look up and down, and one side to the other • Visual field check	Not applicable	• Scan the retina • Auscultate the carotid arteries • Palpate (various)
2	Seated, with legs extended along length of table	Spine	• Rotate shoulders and trunk to each side • Touch toes, with back arched	Not applicable	• Inspect spine
		Posterior chest	Not applicable	Not applicable	• Percuss and auscultate
		Jugular veins	Not applicable	Not applicable	• Assess height of jugular veins
3	Semi-reclined, at about 40 degrees	Anterior chest	Not applicable	Not applicable	• Inspect, percuss, auscultate, palpate (various)
		Heart	Not applicable	Not applicable	• Locate/check cardiac apical impulse • Palpate the precordium • Auscultate
		Abdomen	Not applicable	Not applicable	• Inspect • Palpate and auscultate (various)
4	Lying supine	Lower extremities	• Knees to chest • Heel to buttock, drop knee laterally • Move heel along shin of opposite leg	• Quadriceps • Achilles • Plantar	• Test for tone and power • Test for sense of touch

Illustrated Medical Syndromes

"He who studies medicine without book sails an uncharted sea, but he who studies medicine without patients does not go to sea at all."

—*Sir William Osler*

Illustrated Medical Syndromes

Patient rounds are increasingly conducted in hallways, in conference rooms, and around computer terminals, providing less opportunity for observing and reviewing the clinical signs of medical syndromes. Knowing how to perform exam maneuvers alone will not lead to effective clinical diagnosis. The competent diagnostician will make an effort to become familiar with the clinical signs of medical syndromes.

As an aid to diagnosis, a compendium of medical syndromes is provided in this manual. Each syndrome comprises a list of clinical signs complemented on the facing page with an annotated illustration. (A picture is worth a thousand words!) To facilitate engagement, an open-ended question is posed with each illustration. The syndromes selected for inclusion are ones characterized by clusters of potential signs. It is a limited series, but you are encouraged to develop some of your own syndromes using the blank pages and illustrations provided.

Although eponymous terms are not essential (and may be discouraged by some), they are included for historical interest. They serve not only as a tribute to those named but also as testimony to the power of clinical observation during times when there was not the array of special tests that are available today.

The syndromes are presented as classically described and may be used as a point of reference for evidence-based review. Although it is now less common than in the past to encounter patients presenting with all the potential signs of a particular syndrome—for example, atherosclerotic aortic regurgitation does not display the dramatic "full-house" clinical signs (and eponyms!) encountered with aortic regurgitation associated with syphilis—global migration of persons from less-developed countries may lead to a resurgence of this.

> **PRACTICE POINT: Review the list of clinical signs and study the matching illustration.**
>
> Sketch a patient figure, visualize the illustration, and annotate your sketch. Importantly, develop a habit of reviewing the potential clinical signs of medical conditions you encounter. Use the blank text pages with matching blank figures to add additional medical syndromes of your choosing.

CARDIOLOGY

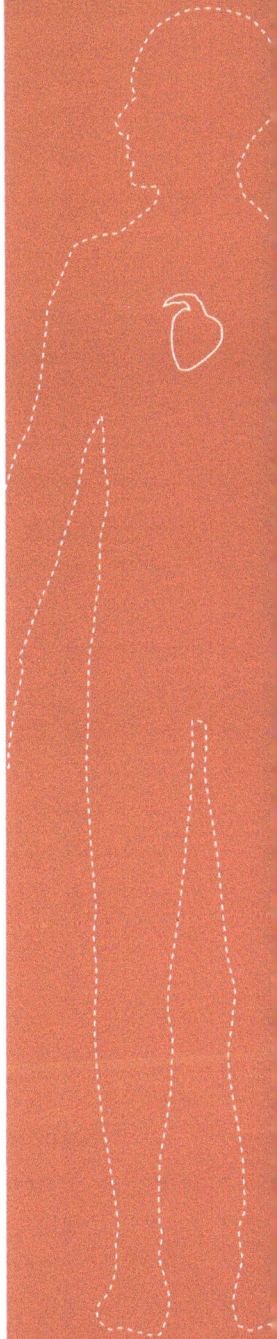

Aortic Regurgitation

Head and Neck

- bobbing of head (de Musset sign)
- pulsation of larynx (Oliver-Cardarelli sign)

Ocular

- retinal artery pulsation (Becker sign)

Oral

- pulsation of uvula (Müller sign)

Integumentary

- flushing and blanching of face and forehead, synchronous with heartbeat (lighthouse sign)
- flushing and blanching of nail bed upon light pressure on end of nail (Quincke sign)

Cardiac

- enlarged heart with sustained apical impulse
- S3 gallop
- to-and-fro murmur: aortic decrescendo diastolic blowing murmur alternating with systolic ejection murmur
- apical diastolic rumbling murmur (Austin Flint murmur)

Arterial

- wide pulse pressure
- popliteal pressure >60 mmHg over brachial pressure (Hill sign)
- collapsing, water hammer pulse (Corrigan pulse)
- pistol shot sounds on auscultation over large arteries – brachial, femoral
- to-and-fro murmur with firm stethoscope pressure over large arteries (Duroziez murmur)

Abdominal

- systolic liver pulsation (Rosenbach sign)
- splenic pulsation (Sailer sign)

Aortic Regurgitation

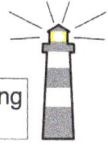

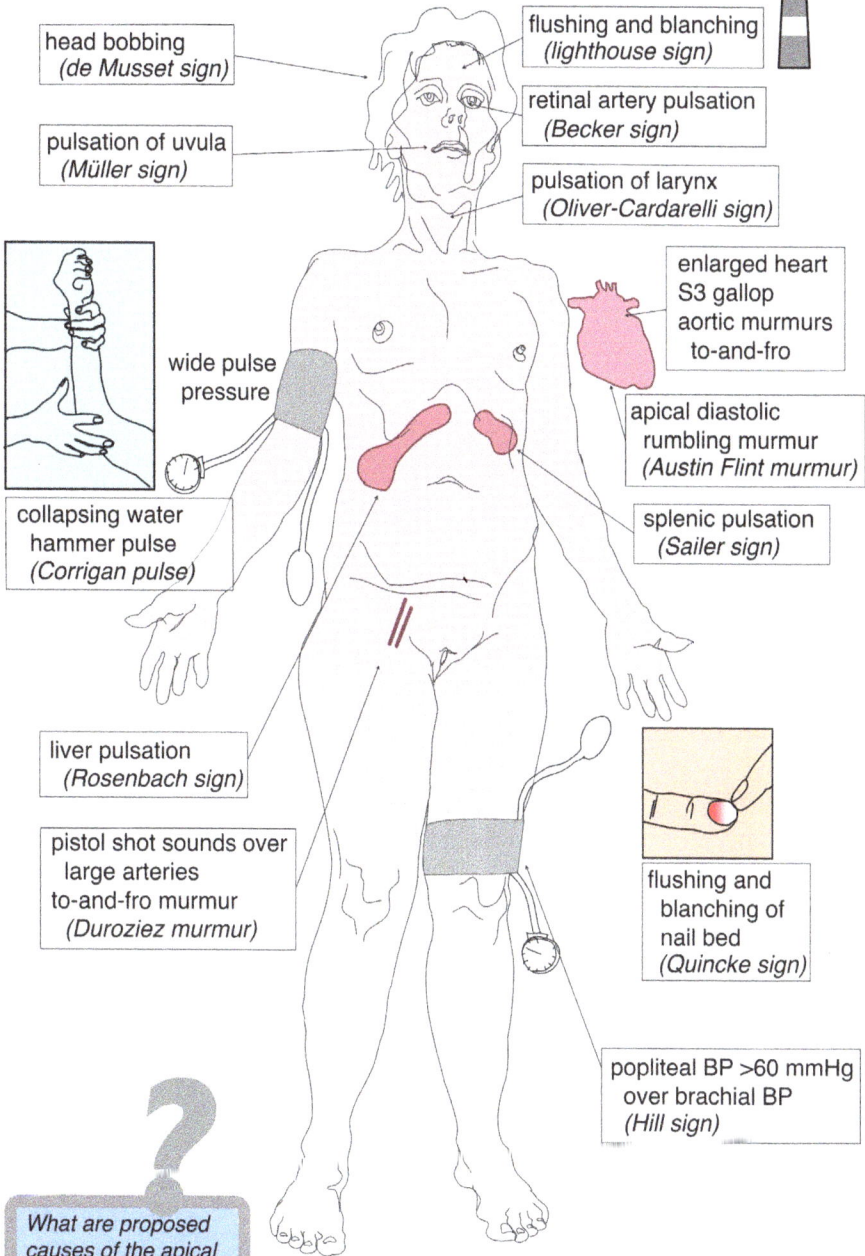

head bobbing
(de Musset sign)

flushing and blanching
(lighthouse sign)

pulsation of uvula
(Müller sign)

retinal artery pulsation
(Becker sign)

pulsation of larynx
(Oliver-Cardarelli sign)

enlarged heart
S3 gallop
aortic murmurs
to-and-fro

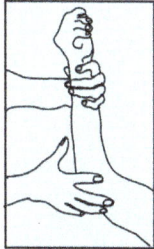

wide pulse
pressure

apical diastolic
rumbling murmur
(Austin Flint murmur)

collapsing water
hammer pulse
(Corrigan pulse)

splenic pulsation
(Sailer sign)

liver pulsation
(Rosenbach sign)

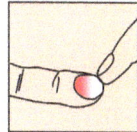

pistol shot sounds over
large arteries
to-and-fro murmur
(Duroziez murmur)

flushing and
blanching of
nail bed
(Quincke sign)

popliteal BP >60 mmHg
over brachial BP
(Hill sign)

What are proposed
causes of the apical
diastolic rumbling
murmur?

Aortic Stenosis (AS)

Cardiac

- exertional angina
- palpable thrill at right second intercostal space
- aortic valve crescendo-decrescendo harsh systolic murmur
  - at right second parasternal intercostal space, +/– palpable thrill
  - radiating to*
    * right midclavicular area and right carotid artery, and left when more severe
    * left sternal border
    * cardiac apex, where it may mimic mitral regurgitation
    * top of skull and right elbow (historically, with severe rheumatic AS)
- diminished S2, +/– paradoxical split
- S4
- sustained apical impulse

Pulmonary

- exertional dyspnea

Venous

- prominent jugular vein a-wave (Bernheim phenomenon)

Arterial

- pulsus parvus et tardus: low volume and delayed upstroke of carotid pulse
- apical-carotid delay: delay between apical impulse and carotid artery
- possible diminished pulse pressure

Neurologic

- episodic cardiac syncope

Picture a sash draped across the right shoulder and across the anterior chest and cardiac apex: the murmur is audible obliquely along the line of the sash.

Aortic Stenosis (AS)

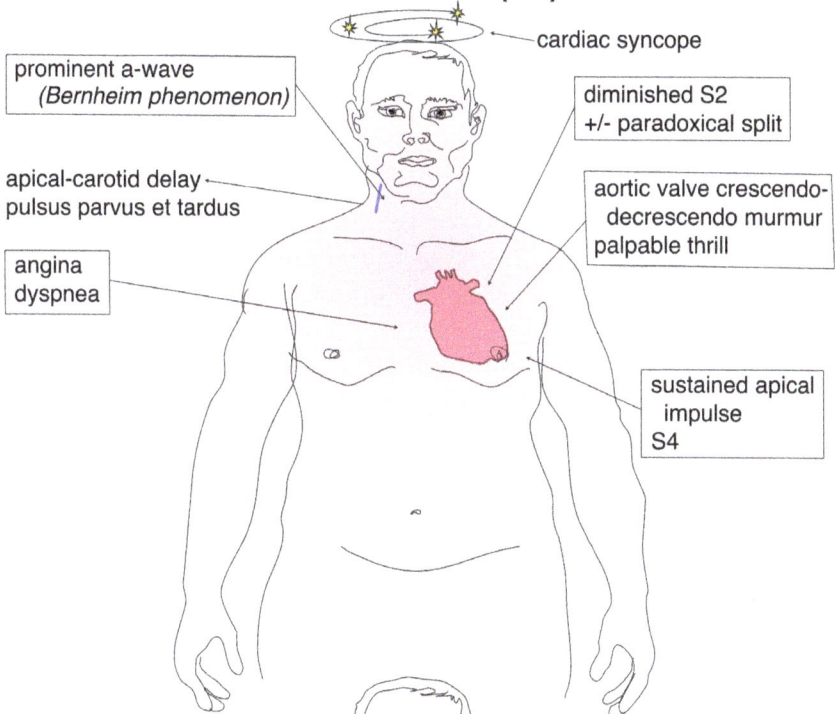

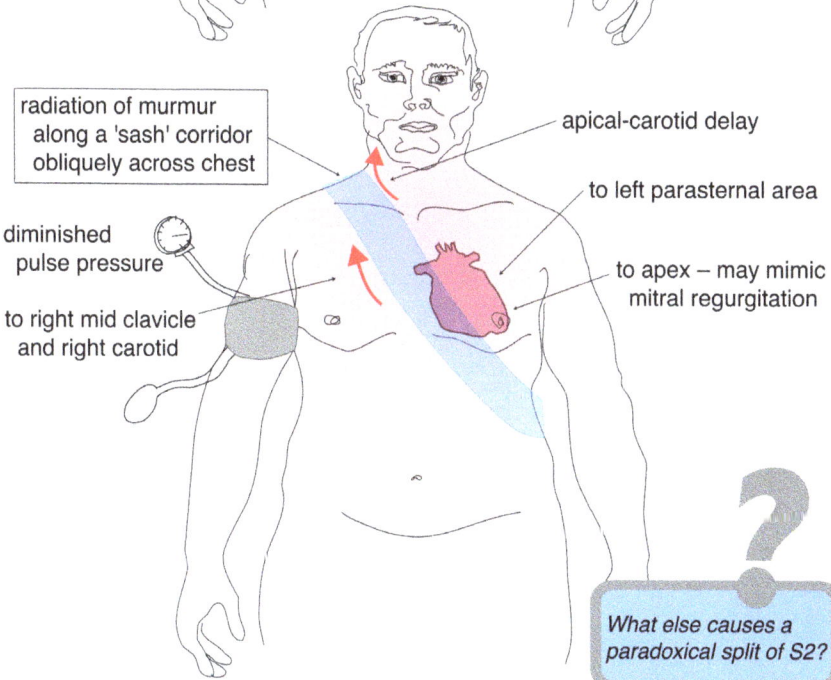

cardiac syncope

prominent a-wave
(Bernheim phenomenon)

diminished S2
+/- paradoxical split

apical-carotid delay
pulsus parvus et tardus

aortic valve crescendo-
decrescendo murmur
palpable thrill

angina
dyspnea

sustained apical
impulse
S4

radiation of murmur
along a 'sash' corridor
obliquely across chest

apical-carotid delay

to left parasternal area

diminished
pulse pressure

to apex – may mimic
mitral regurgitation

to right mid clavicle
and right carotid

What else causes a
paradoxical split of S2?

Signs of congestive heart failure may be a combination of right and left heart failure signs.

Right Heart Failure	Left Heart Failure
• jugular veins elevated	• orthopnea
• Kussmaul sign	• Cheyne-Stokes breathing
• positive hepatojugular reflux (HJR)	• narrow pulse pressure, pulsus alternans
• left parasternal lift	• tachycardia
• right ventricular S3	• lung crackles, wheezing
• +/– tricuspid regurgitation	• laterally displaced cardiac apex
• right side or bilateral pleural effusion	• sustained apical impulse
• hepatomegaly +/– pulsatile liver	• audible S3, S4 may be palpable
• ascites	• mitral or aortic valve bruits
• dependent edema – presacral, pedal	

Congestive Heart Failure (CHF)

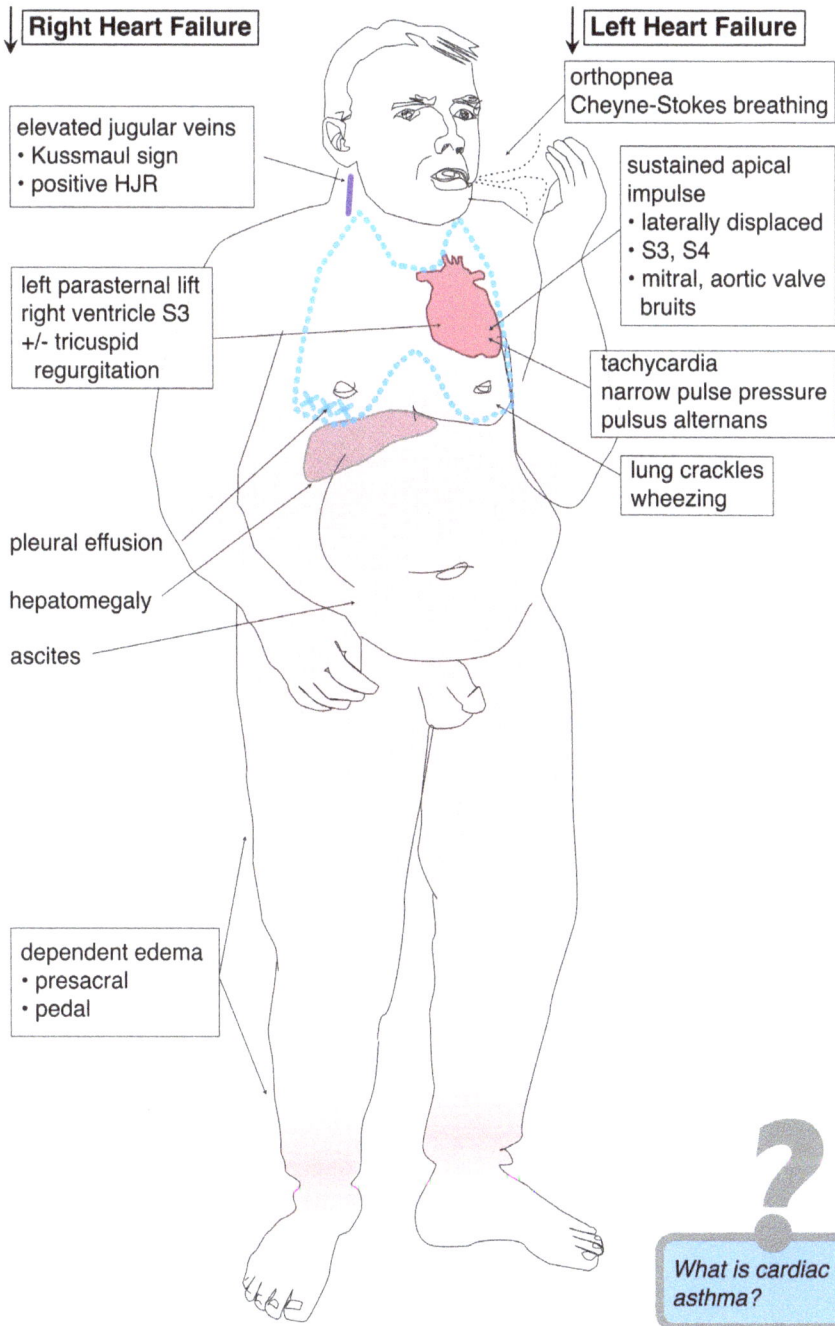

Right Heart Failure

Left Heart Failure

orthopnea
Cheyne-Stokes breathing

elevated jugular veins
• Kussmaul sign
• positive HJR

sustained apical
impulse
• laterally displaced
• S3, S4
• mitral, aortic valve
  bruits

left parasternal lift
right ventricle S3
+/- tricuspid
  regurgitation

tachycardia
narrow pulse pressure
pulsus alternans

lung crackles
wheezing

pleural effusion

hepatomegaly

ascites

dependent edema
• presacral
• pedal

*What is cardiac
asthma?*

Constrictive Pericarditis

Cardiac

- systolic retraction of cardiac apex
- pericardial knock (Beck sign)
- pericardial rub

Venous

- elevated jugular veins
- paradoxical rise during inspiration (Kussmaul sign)
- prominent y-descent (Friedreich sign)

Arterial

- pulsus paradoxus, mild and infrequent

Abdominal

- distention with ascites
- hepatomegaly +/− Pick pseudo-cirrhosis

Extremities

- dependent edema

Constrictive Pericarditis

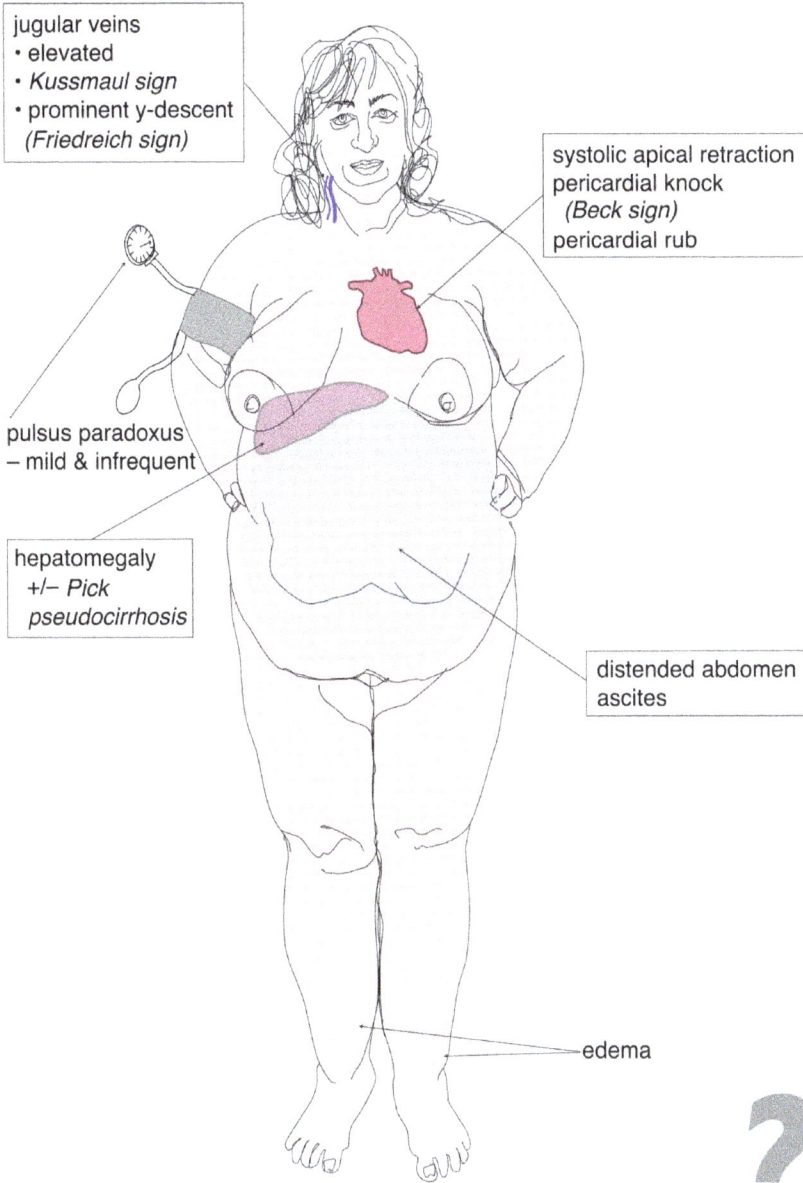

jugular veins
- elevated
- *Kussmaul sign*
- prominent y-descent
  (Friedreich sign)

systolic apical retraction
pericardial knock
  (Beck sign)
pericardial rub

pulsus paradoxus
– mild & infrequent

hepatomegaly
+/– *Pick*
  pseudocirrhosis

distended abdomen
ascites

edema

What causes the pericardial knock?

Pericardial Tamponade

Cardiopulmonary
- point of maximal impulse (PMI)
  - absence of observable PMI
  - detection of PMI obscured on palpation (possible)
  - percussive dullness lateral to PMI (possible)
- percussive dullness at:
  - lower half of sternum (Dressler sign)
  - right parasternal area (Rotch sign)
  - cardiohepatic angle at fifth right intercostal space (Ebstein sign)
  - parasternal second intercostal spaces (ICS)
- posterior left lower chest, +/– bronchial breathing (Ewart sign)

Venous
- elevated jugular veins
- paradoxical rise during inspiration (Kussmaul sign)
- absent y-descent
- positive hepatojugular reflux (HJR)
- peripheral edema

Arterial
- hypotension
- pulsus paradoxus

Abdominal
- hepatomegaly
- epigastric bulging (Auenbrugger sign)

> **Beck triad:**
> - hypotension
> - elevated neck veins
> - muffled heart sounds

Pericardial Tamponade

neck veins
- elevated
- *Kussmaul sign*
- absent y-descent
- positive hepatojugular reflux

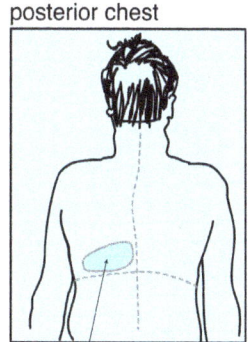

posterior chest

percussive dullness
+/- bronchial breathing
(Ewart sign)

hypotension
pulsus paradoxus

hepatomegaly
epigastric bulging
(Auenbrugger sign)

point of maximal impulse (PMI)
- absent on inspection
- obscured on palpation
- dullness lateral to PMI

muffled heart sounds
percussive dullness:

Beck triad
- hypotension
- elevated neck veins
- muffled heart sounds

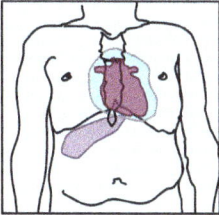

at lower half of sternum
(Dressler sign)
at cardio-hepatic angle
(Ebstein sign)
at right parasternal area
(Rotch sign)
at parasternal second ICS's

edema

How does Ewart sign come about?

General

- febrile
- weight loss

Ocular

- conjunctival hemorrhages
- retinal Roth spots: round or flame-shaped areas of hemorrhage with pale center
- retinal hemorrhages

Cardiac

- cardiac murmur
  - new murmur
  - change in existing murmur
- heart failure

Pulmonary

- pleuritic pain
- pulmonary embolism

Abdominal

- splenomegaly
- splenic rub with infarction

Integumentary

- petechiae – skin and mucous membranes
- embolic infarction
- Osler nodes: small, nodular, painful lesions on pulp of digits or thenar eminence
- Janeway lesions: hemorrhagic, painless macules on palmar or plantar areas
- splinter hemorrhages in nail bed – linear red-brown streaks (usually proximally)
- finger clubbing (Schamroth sign): obliteration of the triangular ("diamond-shaped") window between the bases of the nails when corresponding nails of opposite hands are placed together

Musculoskeletal

- arthritis
- hypertrophic osteoarthropathy

Neurologic

- embolic cerebrovascular accident
- subarachnoid hemorrhage due to mycotic aneurysm

Endocarditis
Subacute Bacterial Endocarditis (SBE)

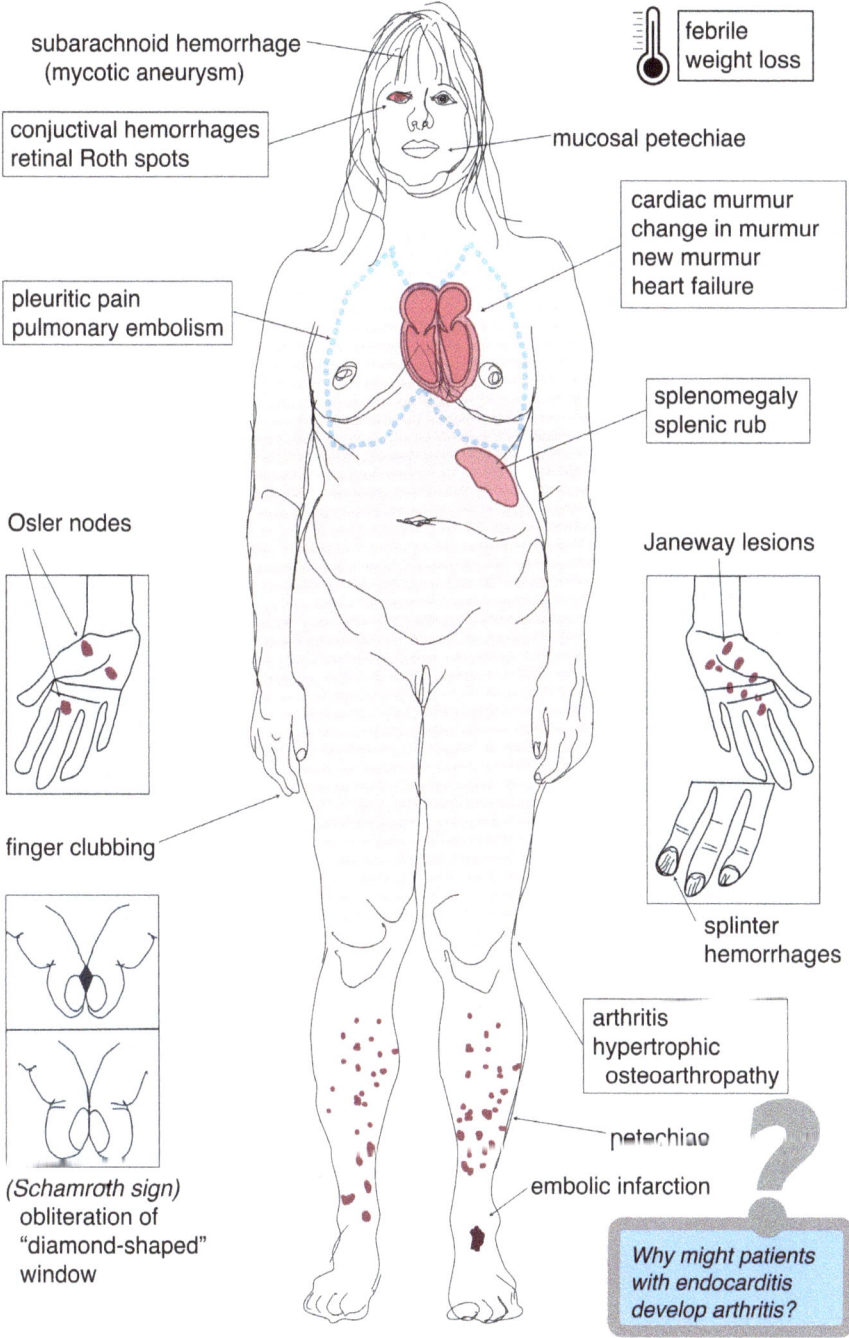

subarachnoid hemorrhage (mycotic aneurysm)

febrile
weight loss

conjuctival hemorrhages
retinal Roth spots

mucosal petechiae

cardiac murmur
change in murmur
new murmur
heart failure

pleuritic pain
pulmonary embolism

splenomegaly
splenic rub

Osler nodes

Janeway lesions

finger clubbing

splinter
hemorrhages

arthritis
hypertrophic
osteoarthropathy

petechiae

embolic infarction

(Schamroth sign)
obliteration of
"diamond-shaped"
window

?

*Why might patients
with endocarditis
develop arthritis?*

ENDOCRINOLOGY

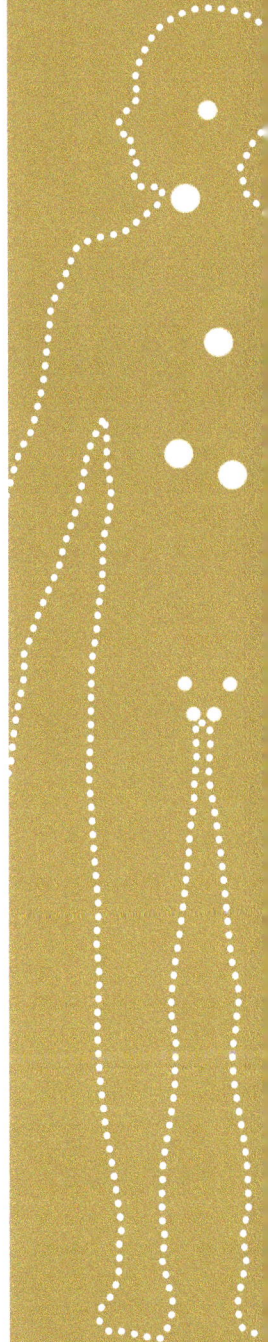

Acromegaly

Facial

- coarse features
- deep creases on forehead and nasolabial fold
- thick eyelids
- broad nose
- thick lips
- macroglossia

Integumentary

- acanthosis nigricans
- hyperpigmentation
- hypertrichosis
- fibromas

Cardiac

- left ventricular hypertrophy
- mitral regurgitation

Arterial

- hypertension

Abdominal

- hepatomegaly
- splenomegaly

Musculoskeletal

- proximal myopathy
- large hands and feet, increased soft tissue

Endocrine

- goiter

Neurologic

- carpal tunnel syndrome

Gigantism: This condition occurs when hypersecretion of insulin-like growth factor 1 (IGF-1) occurs during childhood, before the bone epiphyses fuse. In addition to the features of acromegaly, other features might include tall stature, skull frontal bossing, and visual field defects.

Acromegaly

coarse facial features
- deep creases
- thick eyelids
- broad nose
- thick lips

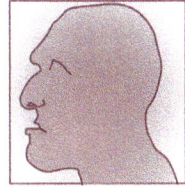

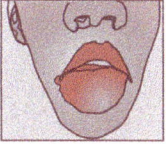

macroglossia

prognathism

goiter

left ventricular hypertrophy
mitral regurgitation

acanthosis nigricans

hyperpigmentation

hypertrichosis

fibromas

hypertension

hepatomegaly
splenomegaly

carpal tunnel
syndrome

large hands

proximal myopathy

large feet

What is McCune-
Albright syndrome?

Cushing's Disease

Body Habitus

- redistribution of fat
  - moon face
  - buffalo hump
  - supraclavicular fat pads
  - centripetal obesity

Integumentary

- plethoric face
- lanugo facial hair
- thin skin ("cigarette paper" appearance)
- purple striae
- ecchymoses
- acanthosis nigricans
- acne
- slow wound healing
- hirsutism (females)

Cardiac

- left ventricular hypertrophy

Arterial

- hypertension

Musculoskeletal

- proximal myopathy
- muscle wasting of extremities
- bone fractures
- avascular necrosis (joints)

Extremities

- pedal edema

Neuropsychiatric

- depression
- emotional lability

Cushing's Disease

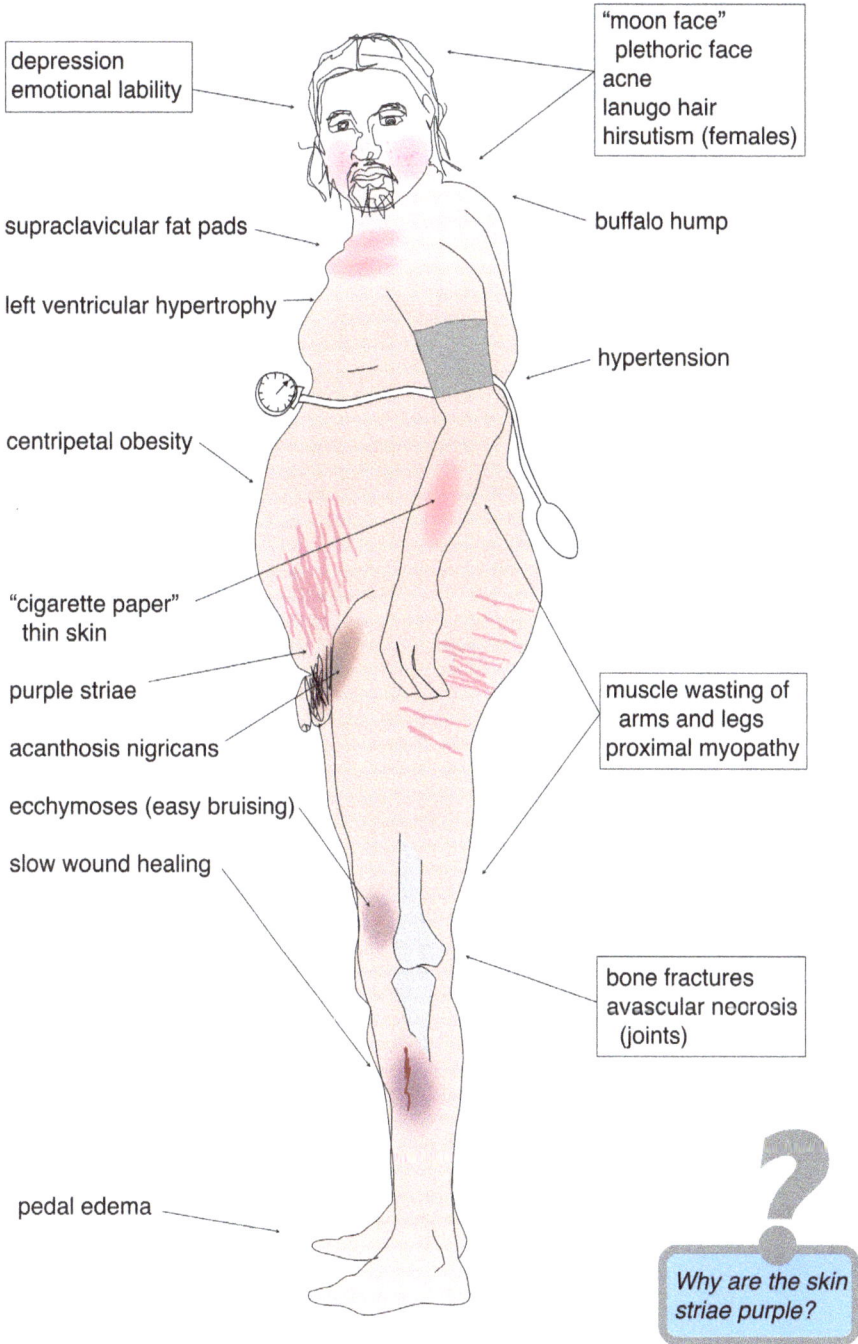

depression
emotional lability

"moon face"
 plethoric face
acne
lanugo hair
hirsutism (females)

supraclavicular fat pads

buffalo hump

left ventricular hypertrophy

hypertension

centripetal obesity

"cigarette paper"
 thin skin

purple striae

acanthosis nigricans

muscle wasting of
 arms and legs
proximal myopathy

ecchymoses (easy bruising)

slow wound healing

bone fractures
avascular necrosis
 (joints)

pedal edema

Why are the skin
striae purple?

Diabetes Mellitus Complications

Ocular

- retinopathy
- cataracts
- glaucoma
- blindness

Oral

- periodontal disease

Integumentary

- dry skin*
- infections, bacterial and fungal
- acanthosis nigricans
- diabetic dermopathy
- necrobiosis lipoidica diabeticorum
- digital sclerosis
- eruptive xanthomas
- ischemic ulcers

Cardiac

- coronary artery disease
- diabetic cardiomyopathy

Vascular

- hypertension
- orthostatic hypotension*
- peripheral vascular disease (PVD)
- gangrene, amputations

Abdominal

- gastroparesis, gut dysmotility*
- hepatomegaly, fatty liver

Renal

- chronic kidney disease signs
- edema

Genitourinary

- erectile dysfunction*

Musculoskeletal

- diabetic myonecrosis
- Charcot arthropathy

Neurologic

- strokes, transient ischemic attacks (TIAs)
- cognitive impairment
- peripheral neuropathy and mononeuropathies
- diabetic amyotrophy (proximal diabetic neuropathy)
- *autonomic neuropathies (indicated above)

Diabetes Mellitus Complications

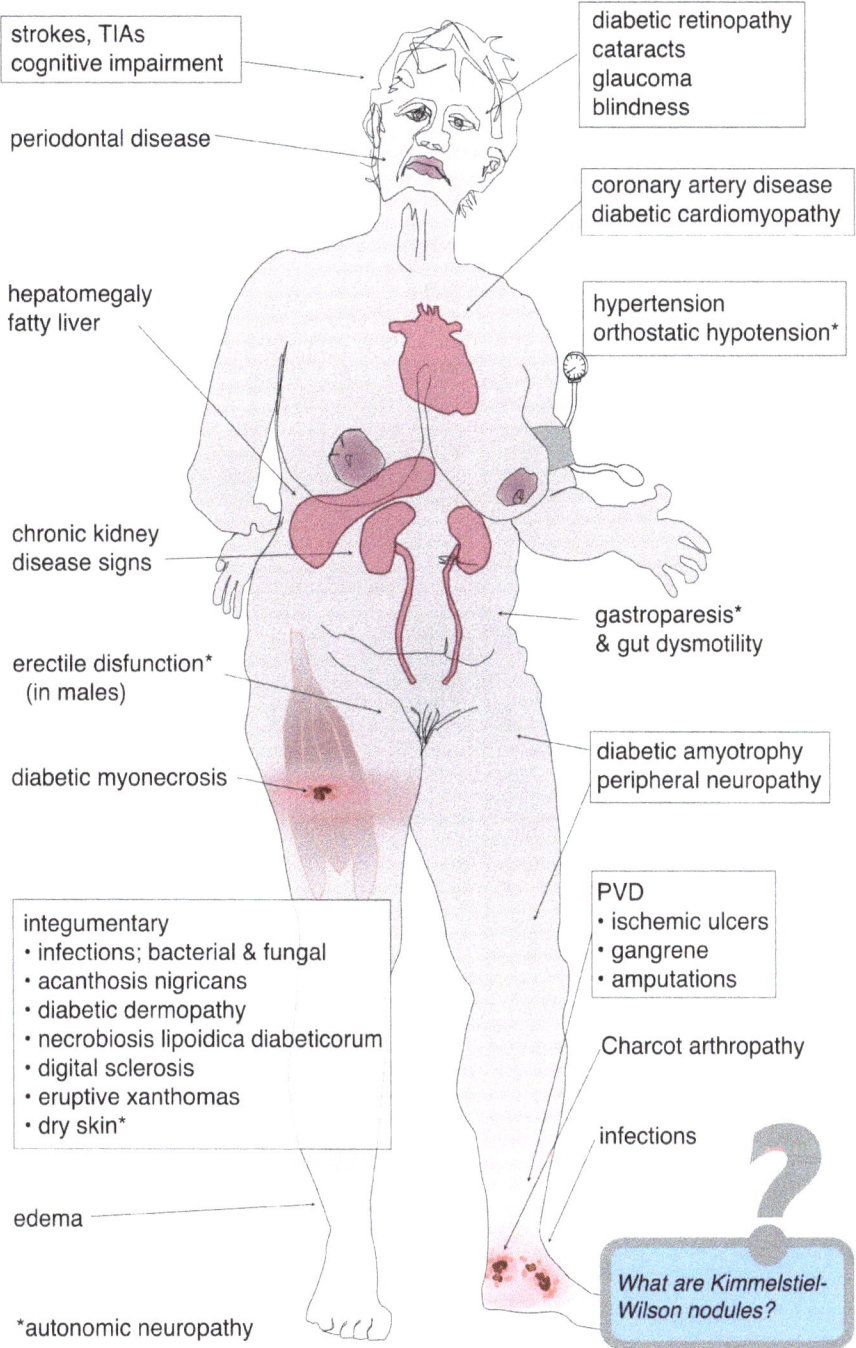

strokes, TIAs
cognitive impairment

periodontal disease

diabetic retinopathy
cataracts
glaucoma
blindness

coronary artery disease
diabetic cardiomyopathy

hepatomegaly
fatty liver

hypertension
orthostatic hypotension*

chronic kidney
disease signs

gastroparesis*
& gut dysmotility

erectile disfunction*
(in males)

diabetic myonecrosis

diabetic amyotrophy
peripheral neuropathy

PVD
• ischemic ulcers
• gangrene
• amputations

integumentary
• infections; bacterial & fungal
• acanthosis nigricans
• diabetic dermopathy
• necrobiosis lipoidica diabeticorum
• digital sclerosis
• eruptive xanthomas
• dry skin*

Charcot arthropathy

infections

edema

*autonomic neuropathy

? What are Kimmelstiel-
Wilson nodules?

Hyperthyroidism due to Graves Disease

General

- restlessness
- weight loss

Endocrine

- goiter, smooth and symmetrical
- thyroid bruit

Integumentary

- warm, moist skin
- onycholysis (Plummer sign): thinning of nails, lifting off from nail bed
- pretibial myxedema (an infiltrative dermopathy)

Extremities

- thyroid acropachy: digital soft tissue swelling, finger clubbing, periosteal reaction

Ocular

- lid lag (von Graefe sign): white sclera visible above cornea during downward movement of eye
- lid retraction (Dalrymple sign): widening of palpebral opening, white sclera visible between retracted upper eyelid and cornea (thyroid stare)
- thyroid ophthalmopathy
  - exophthalmos (anterior protrusion of the orbit)
  - diplopia and limitation of eye movement
  - conjunctival chemosis (edema) and hyperemia

Cardiac

- tachycardia +/– atrial fibrillation
- cardiac flow murmur
- scratchy rub or murmur (Means-Lerman scratch)

Arterial

- systolic hypertension

Musculoskeletal

- proximal muscle weakness

Neurologic

- fine tremor of hands
- brisk tendon reflexes

Hyperthyroidism due to Graves Disease

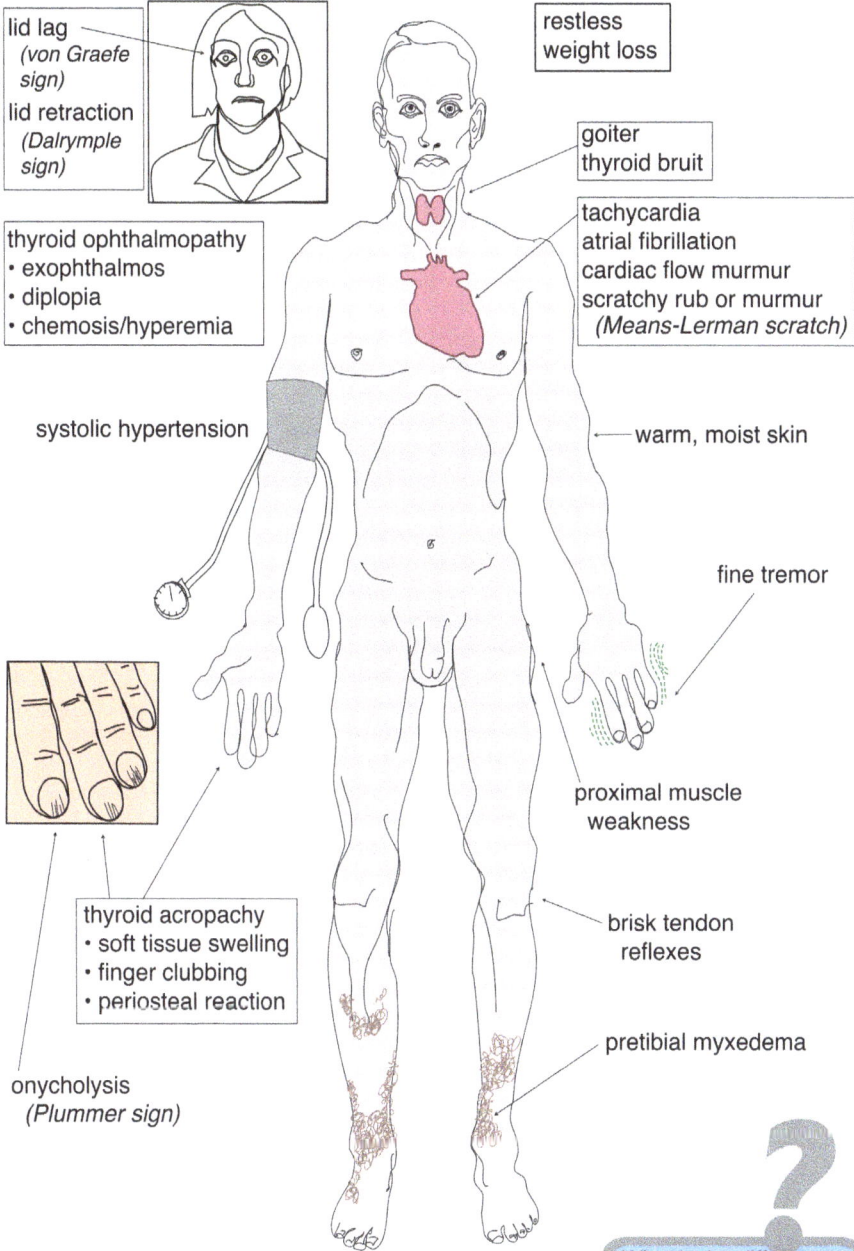

lid lag
(von Graefe sign)

lid retraction
(Dalrymple sign)

thyroid ophthalmopathy
• exophthalmos
• diplopia
• chemosis/hyperemia

systolic hypertension

thyroid acropachy
• soft tissue swelling
• finger clubbing
• periosteal reaction

onycholysis
(Plummer sign)

restless
weight loss

goiter
thyroid bruit

tachycardia
atrial fibrillation
cardiac flow murmur
scratchy rub or murmur
(Means-Lerman scratch)

warm, moist skin

fine tremor

proximal muscle
weakness

brisk tendon
reflexes

pretibial myxedema

What is the difference between exophthalmos and proptosis?

Hypothyroidism

General

- weight gain
- slow movement
- slow speech
- cool extremities
- jaundice

Endocrine

- goiter

Facial

- coarse features
- puffy eyes
- loss of temporal portion of eyebrows
- pasty complexion

Oropharyngeal

- macroglossia
- hoarse voice

Auditory

- decreased hearing

Integumentary

- cool, dry skin
- non-pitting edema (myxedema)

Cardiac

- bradycardia
- pericardial effusion

Arterial

- hypotension

Abdominal

- ascites (uncommon)

Neuropsychiatric

- hyporeflexia with delayed relaxation phase
- carpal tunnel syndrome
- depression
- emotional lability

Myxedema coma:

- altered mental state
- coma
- hypothermia
- depressed respiration
- hypotension
- marked bradycardia
- cardiogenic shock

Hypothyroidism

weight gain
slow movement
cool extremities
jaundice

decreased hearing

slow speech
hoarse voice
macroglossia

goiter

jaundice

ascites
  (uncommon)

depression
emotional lability

coarse features
pasty complexion
puffy eyes
loss of temporal
  portion of eyebrows

pericardial effusion
hypotension
bradycardia

carpal tunnel
  syndrome

cool dry skin

myxedema coma
• altered mental state
• coma
• hypothermia
• depressed respiration
• hypotension
• marked bradycardia
• cardiogenic shock

non-pitting edema
  (myxedema)

hyporeflexia with
  delayed relaxation

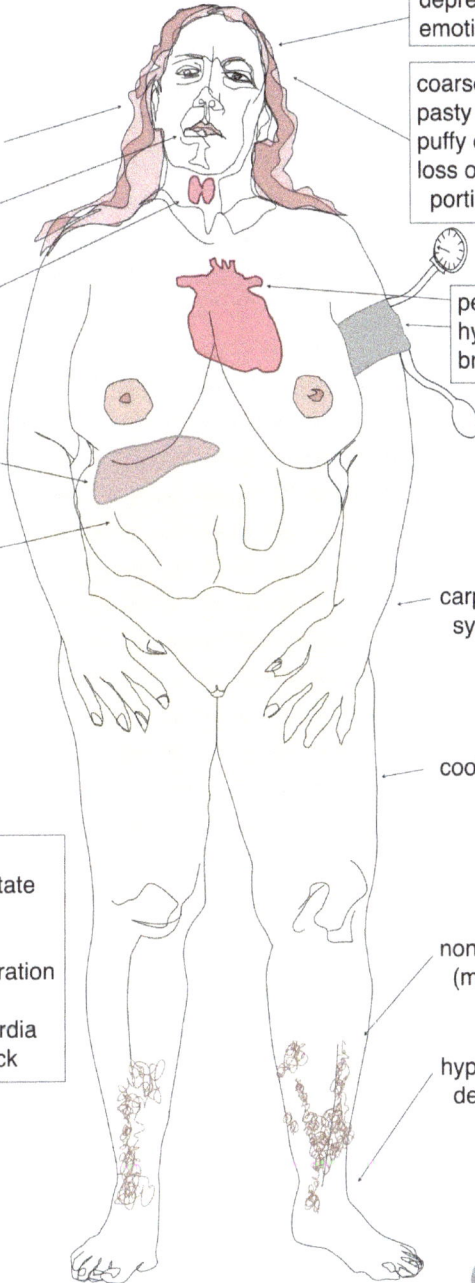

*What is Riedel
thyroiditis?*

Primary Adrenal Insufficiency (Addison's Disease)

General

- weakness
- fatigue
- pallor
- fever
- weight loss

Oral

- buccal mucosa pigmentation

Integumentary

- bronze pigmentation, generalized with darker areas in
  - axillae
  - nipples
  - scars
  - palmar creases
  - sun-exposed areas

- vitiligo
- loss of axillary and pubic hair

Arterial

- postural hypotension

Neurologic

- postural dizziness

Adrenal crisis: above signs, plus
- tachycardia
- dehydration
- hypovolemic shock
- delirium
- vomiting
- acute abdomen

Primary Adrenal Insufficiency
(Addison's Disease)

fever
weakness
fatigue
pallor
weight loss

postural dizziness

buccal mucosa pigmentation

loss of axillary hair

postural hypotension

bronze pigmentation darker areas
• axillae
• nipples
• scars
• palmar creases
• sun exposed

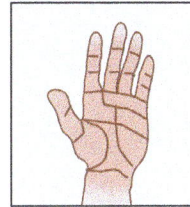

loss of pubic hair

vitiligo

adrenal crisis
• tachycardia
• dehydration
• hypovolemic shock
• delirium
• vomiting
• acute abdomen

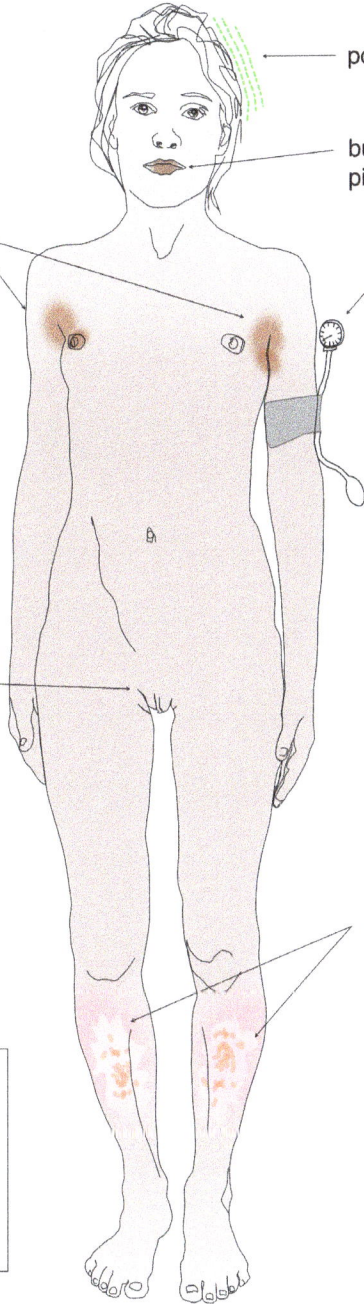

What is Schmidt syndrome?

GASTROENTEROLOGY

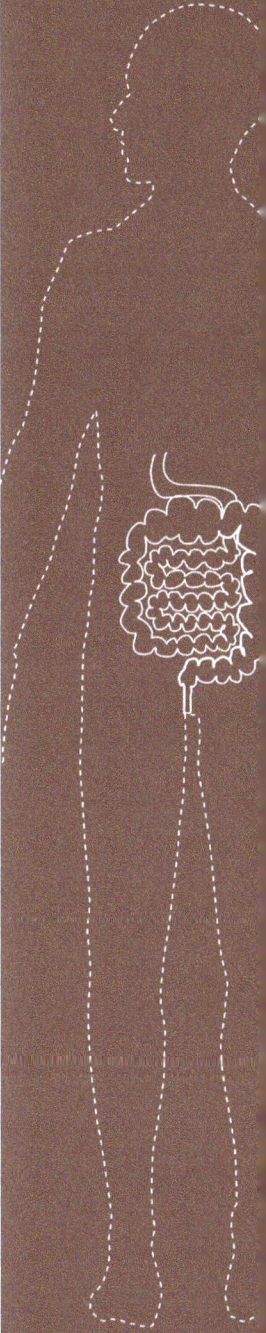

Cirrhosis with Portal Hypertension and Hepatic Failure

General

- weight loss
- muscle atrophy
- jaundice
- fetor hepaticus
- peripheral edema

Integumentary

- spider angiomas (mostly upper trunk and face)
- palmar erythema
- loss of pubic and body hair

Cardiac

- hyperdynamic circulation

Pulmonary

- cyanosis with hepatopulmonary syndrome

Abdominal

- collateral veins radiating from the umbilicus
- caput medusae: dilated umbilical veins reminiscent of a nest of serpents
- venous hum, audible in midline above umbilicus (Cruveilhier-Baumgarten bruit)
- small liver with firm edge
- splenomegaly
- puddle sign*
- ascites with shifting dullness

Endocrine

- gynecomastia
- testicular atrophy

Neurologic

- asterixis (liver flap)
- encephalopathy

*Puddle sign: After lying supine for 5 minutes, the patient rises to hands and knees. Stethoscope is placed on most dependent part of the abdomen and moved slowly laterally while a finger flicks on one flank. The transition from low frequency to higher frequency sound determines the edge of the fluid puddle. The maneuver is of historical interest only, and of no clinical value.

Cirrhosis with Portal Hypertension and Hepatic Failure

weight loss
muscle atrophy
peripheral edema

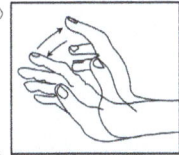

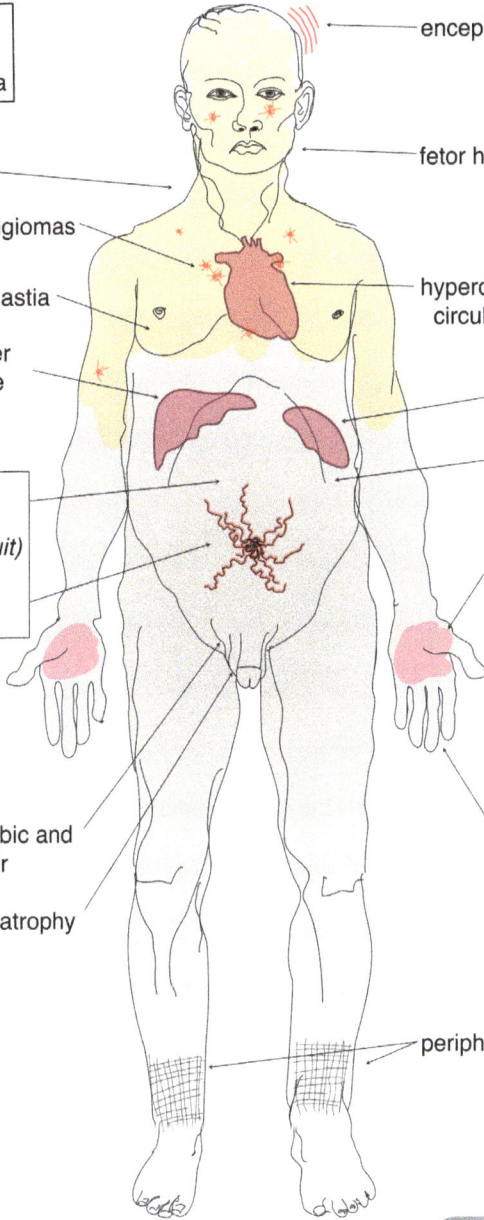

encephalopathy

jaundice

fetor hepaticus

spider angiomas

gynecomastia

hyperdynamic circulation

small liver
firm edge

splenomegaly

ascites with
shifting dullness

venous hum
(Cruveilhier-Baumgarten bruit)

caput medusae
collateral veins

palmar erythema

loss of pubic and
body hair

testicular atrophy

asterixis
(liver flap)

peripheral edema

How does cyanosis in the hepatopulmonary syndrome develop?

Crohn's Disease

General

- intermittent fever
- pallor
- jaundice

Abdominal

- pain and tenderness
- masses, often right lower quadrant
- fistulas and sinuses
- abscesses
- intestinal obstruction
- hepatomegaly (fatty liver, autoimmune hepatitis, sclerosing cholangitis)

Anorectal

- perianal sinuses
- fissures
- abscesses
- rectal prolapse

Genitourinary

- enterovesical fistulas
- enterovaginal fistulas

EXTRAINTESTINAL MANIFESTATIONS

Ocular

- episcleritis
- uveitis

Oral

- aphthous ulcers
- angular stomatitis

Integumentary

- erythema nodosum
- psoriasis
- pyoderma gangrenosum
- vasculitis

Cardiovascular

- pericarditis
- myocarditis (rare)
- deep vein thrombosis

Pulmonary

- pulmonary embolism
- pleuritis

Renal

- renal colic

Musculoskeletal

- ankylosing spondylitis
- sacroiliitis
- digital clubbing
- arthritis

Crohn's Disease

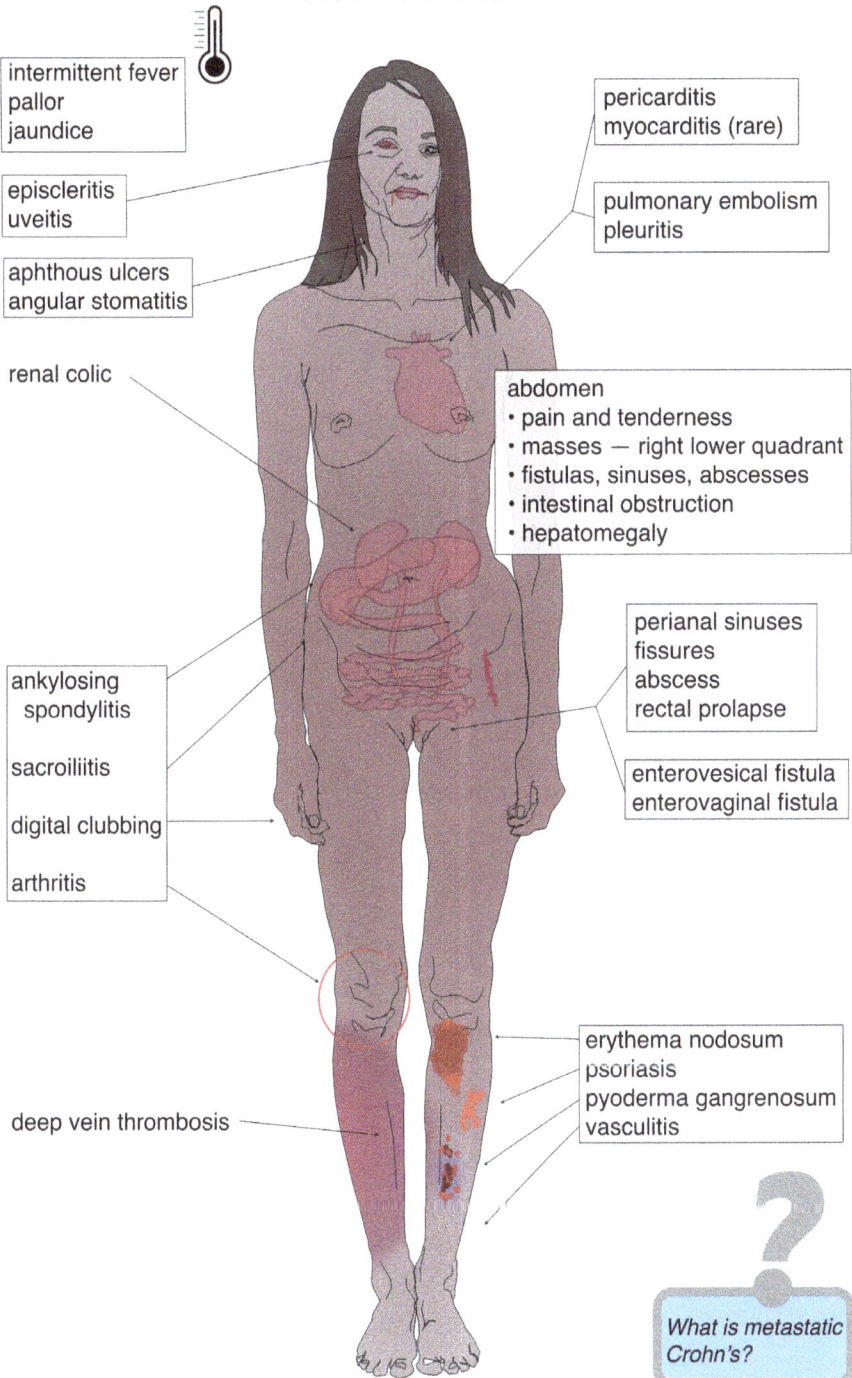

intermittent fever
pallor
jaundice

episcleritis
uveitis

aphthous ulcers
angular stomatitis

renal colic

ankylosing
  spondylitis

sacroiliitis

digital clubbing

arthritis

deep vein thrombosis

pericarditis
myocarditis (rare)

pulmonary embolism
pleuritis

abdomen
• pain and tenderness
• masses — right lower quadrant
• fistulas, sinuses, abscesses
• intestinal obstruction
• hepatomegaly

perianal sinuses
fissures
abscess
rectal prolapse

enterovesical fistula
enterovaginal fistula

erythema nodosum
psoriasis
pyoderma gangrenosum
vasculitis

What is metastatic Crohn's?

Hemochromatosis

Integumentary

- skin bronzing
- hyperpigmentation
- loss of body hair
- koilonychia (spoon nails)

Cardiac

- cardiomegaly
- cardiomyopathy
- congestive heart failure
- abnormal heart sounds
- conduction disturbance

Abdominal

- hepatosplenomegaly
- cirrhosis
- portal hypertension
- liver failure signs

Musculoskeletal

- arthropathies
    - metacarpophalangeal (MCP) joints, second and third
    - proximal interphalangeal (PIP) joints
    - knees, feet, back, neck

Endocrine

- hypothyroidism
- testicular atrophy
- gynecomastia
- diabetes (bronze diabetes)

Hemochromatosis

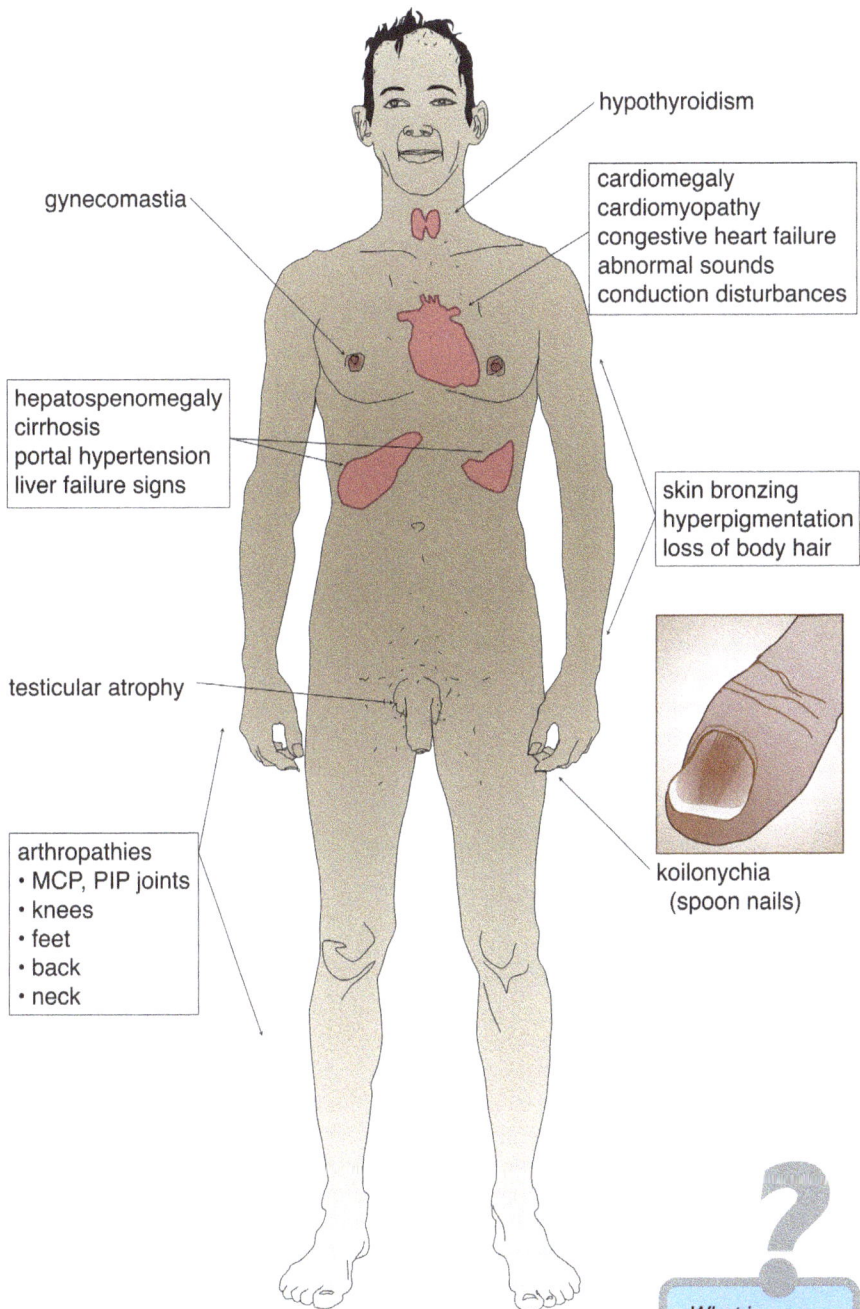

hypothyroidism

cardiomegaly
cardiomyopathy
congestive heart failure
abnormal sounds
conduction disturbances

gynecomastia

hepatospenomegaly
cirrhosis
portal hypertension
liver failure signs

skin bronzing
hyperpigmentation
loss of body hair

testicular atrophy

koilonychia
(spoon nails)

arthropathies
• MCP, PIP joints
• knees
• feet
• back
• neck

What is
hemosiderosis?

Hepatitis C

Most clinical signs occur late, usually with features of chronic liver disease.

Ocular
- keratoconjunctivitis sicca

Integumentary
- porphyria cutanea tarda
  - increased hair growth
  - skin photosensitivity
  - blisters and crusting
- cutaneous necrotizing vasculitis (cryoglobulinemia)
- thrombocytopenic purpura
- Raynaud syndrome
- lichen planus

Hepatic
- chronic liver disease signs (see "Cirrhosis with Portal Hypertension and Hepatic Failure")

Neurologic
- sensory peripheral neuropathy

Autoimmune
- Sjögren syndrome signs (see "Sjögren Syndrome")

Hepatitis C

(most clinical signs occur late)

+/- Chronic Liver Disease Signs   +/- Sjögren Syndrome Signs

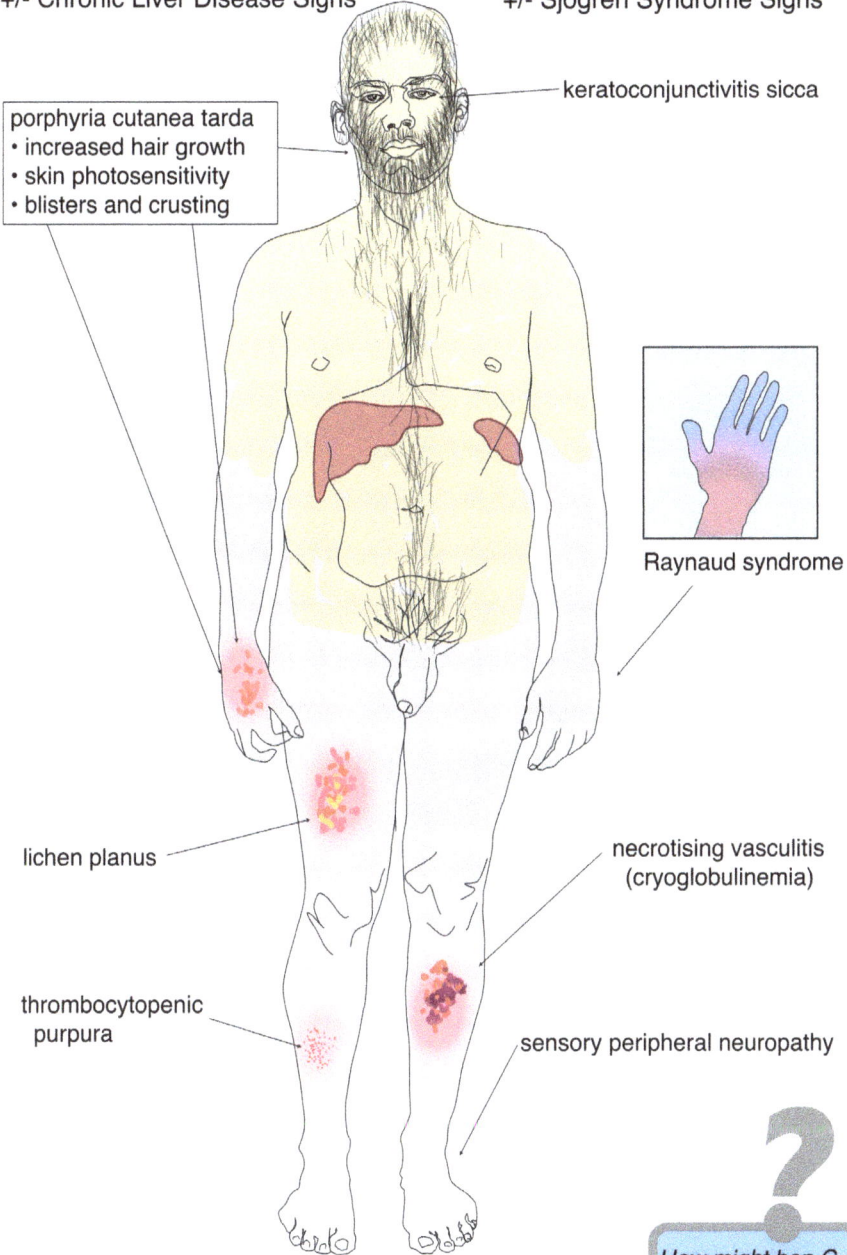

keratoconjunctivitis sicca

porphyria cutanea tarda
• increased hair growth
• skin photosensitivity
• blisters and crusting

Raynaud syndrome

lichen planus

necrotising vasculitis
(cryoglobulinemia)

thrombocytopenic
  purpura

sensory peripheral neuropathy

How might hep C
affect the kidneys?

Primary Biliary Cirrhosis (PBC)

General

- middle-aged female (predominantly)
- fatigue, profound and lasting
- jaundice

Ocular

- xerophthalmia
- xanthelasma

Oral

- xerostomia

Integumentary

- hyperpigmentation
- pruritis
- excoriations

Abdominal

- hepatomegaly, painful
- splenomegaly

Late-stage PBC: chronic liver disease signs (see "Cirrhosis with Portal Hypertension and Hepatic Failure")

Associated conditions:

- Sjögren syndrome (see "Sjögren Syndrome")
- scleroderma (see "Scleroderma")
- rheumatoid arthritis (see "Rheumatoid Arthritis")
- renal tubular acidosis
- autoimmune thyroiditis
- lichen planus
- discoid lupus

Primary Biliary Cirrhosis (PBC)

middle-aged female
fatigue
jaundice

xerophthalmia
xanthelasma

xerostomia

integumentary
• hyperpigmentation
• pruritus
• excoriations

hepatomegaly
— pain

splenomegaly

associated conditions
• Sjögren syndrome
• scleroderma
• rheumatoid arthritis
• renal tubular acidosis
• autoimmune thyroiditis
• lichen planus
• discoid lupus

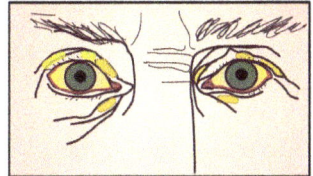

xanthelasma and yellow eyes

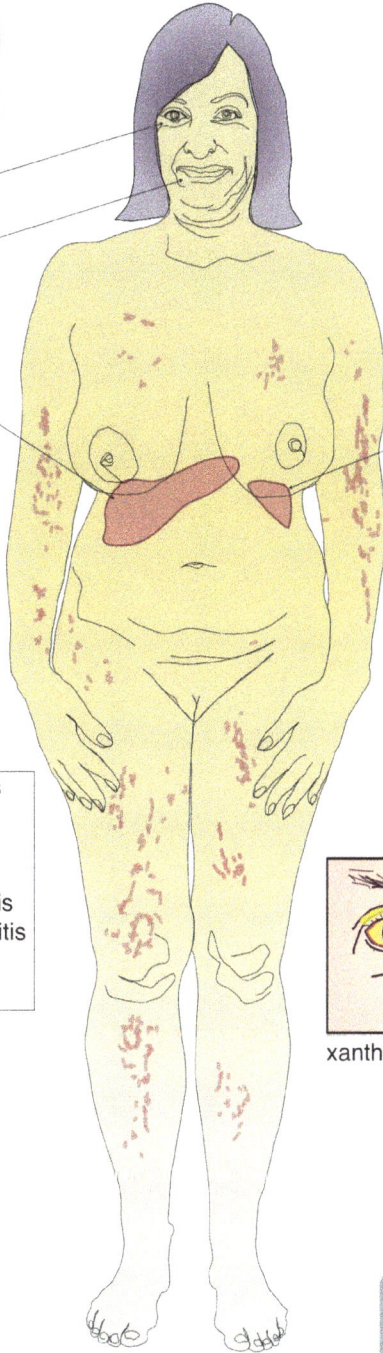

?

Why do patients with PBC suffer from pruritis?

HEMATOLOGY/ ONCOLOGY

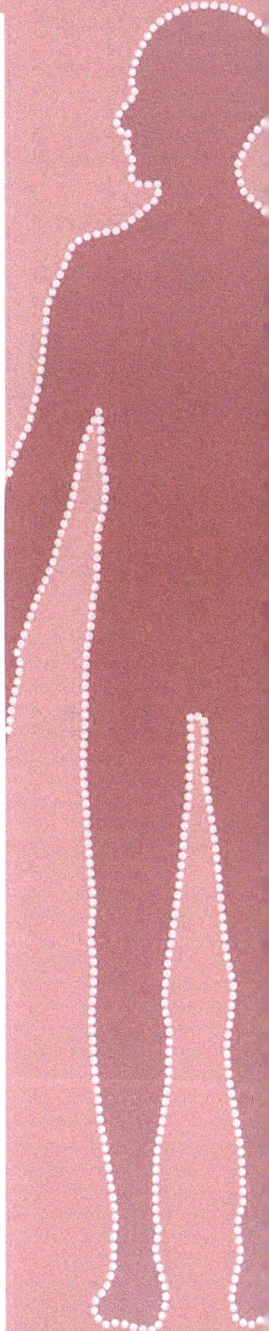

General

- fever
- sweating
- fatigue
- anemia

Lymphatic

- lymphadenopathy

Nasal

- epistaxis

Oral

- gingivitis
- bleeding gums

Integumentary

- purpura
- ecchymoses
- petechial rashes
- leukemia cutis
  - nodules
  - papules
  - plaques

Cardiac

- flow murmurs
- chest pain

Pulmonary

- cough
- dyspnea
- pneumonia

Abdominal

- hepatomegaly
- splenomegaly

Neurologic

- headache
- visual disturbances

Oncologic

- chloroma (myeloid sarcoma)

Leukostasis:

- respiratory distress
- altered mental state
- convulsions
- coma

Acute Myeloid Leukemia (AML)

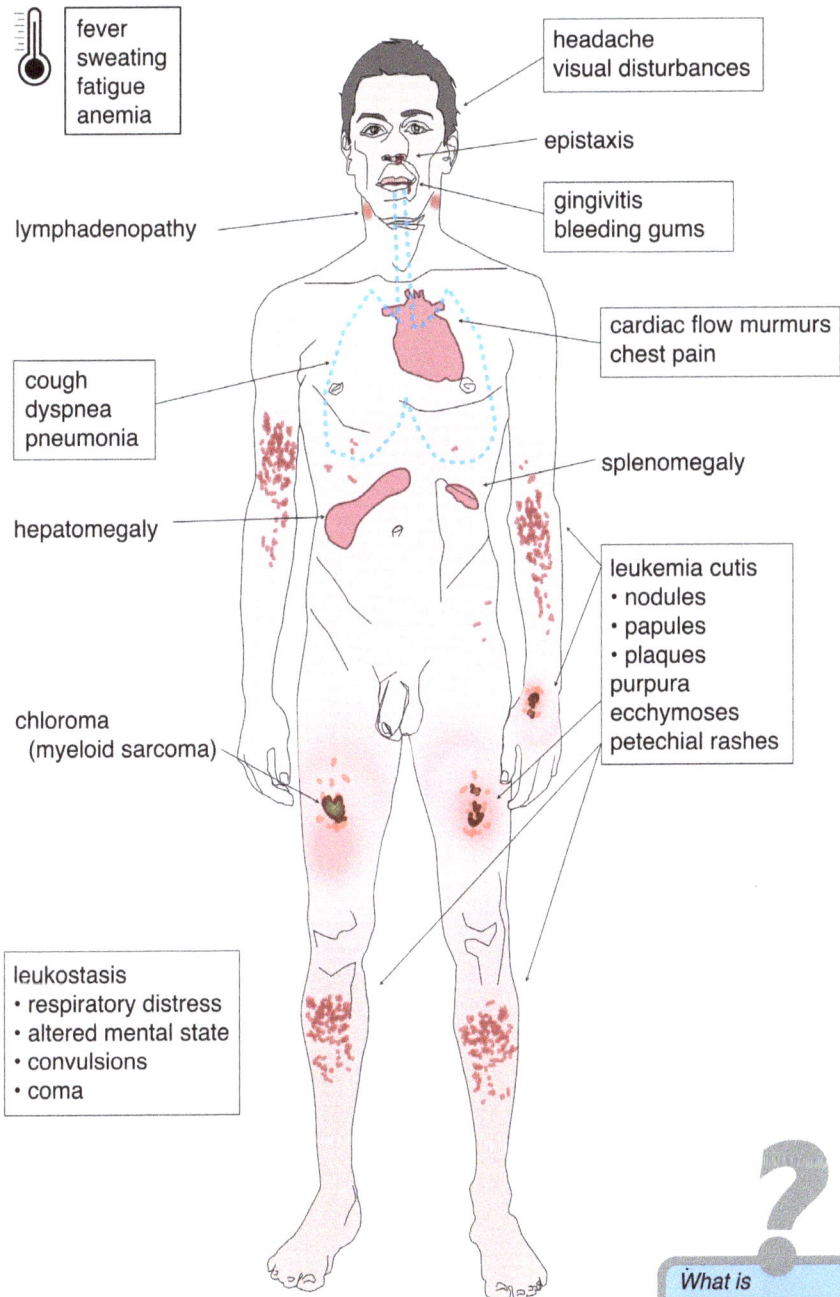

fever
sweating
fatigue
anemia

headache
visual disturbances

epistaxis

gingivitis
bleeding gums

lymphadenopathy

cardiac flow murmurs
chest pain

cough
dyspnea
pneumonia

splenomegaly

hepatomegaly

leukemia cutis
• nodules
• papules
• plaques
purpura
ecchymoses
petechial rashes

chloroma
 (myeloid sarcoma)

leukostasis
• respiratory distress
• altered mental state
• convulsions
• coma

What is
myelodysplastic
syndrome?

Hodgkin Lymphoma

General

- weight loss
- intermittent fever
- Pel-Ebstein fever (rare)

Pharyngeal

- involvement of Waldeyer ring

Lymphatic

- painless lymphadenopathy
  - occipital
  - cervical
  - axillary
  - epitrochlear
  - inguinal
- painful lymphadenopathy – lymph node pain induced by alcohol consumption

Integumentary

- excoriations
- pruritis

Venous

- superior vena cava (SVC) syndrome
  - bluish congestion of face, chest, arms
  - dilated veins

Pulmonary

- cough
- chest pain

Abdominal

- hepatomegaly
- splenomegaly
- distension

Potential associated complications:

- cerebellar degeneration
- Guillain-Barré syndrome
- multifocal leukoencephalopathy

Hodgkin Lymphoma

intermittent fever
Pel-Ebstein fever
weight loss

Waldeyer ring involvement

SVC syndrome
• bluish congestion
• dilated veins

cough
chest pain

painless
lymphadenopathy
• occipatal
• cervical
• axillary
• epitrochlear
• inguinal

hepatomegaly
splenomegaly
abdominal distension

lymph node pain
  induced by alcohol

excoriations
pruritus

potential signs
• cerebellar degeneration
• Guillain-Barré syndrome
• multifocal leukoencephalopathy

What is the pattern
of Pel-Ebstein fever?

Pernicious Anemia

General

- anemia
- low-grade fever
- weight loss

Ocular

- optic neuritis
- retinal hemorrhages

Oral

- beefy red tongue

Integumentary

- lemon-yellow, waxy pallor
- jaundice (mild)

Cardiac

- tachycardia
- congestive heart failure (possible)

Abdominal

- abdominal pain
- nausea, vomiting
- palpable spleen tip (mild splenomegaly)

Urinary

- bladder distension

Neurologic

- sensorimotor peripheral neuropathy
- subacute combined degeneration (SACD) of spinal cord
  - loss of position sense
  - loss of vibration sense
  - ataxia, positive Romberg test
  - spasticity, hyperreflexia
  - weakness, paraplegia
  - Babinski reflex

Neuropsychiatric

- cognitive deficit
- psychiatric disturbances
  - "megaloblastic madness"

Pernicious Anemia

anemia
low-grade fever
weight loss

cognitive deficit
psychiatric disturbances
"megaloblastic madness"

lemon-yellow waxy pallor
jaundice

optic neuritis
retinal hemorrhages

beefy red tongue

subacute combined
degeneration of spinal
cord
• loss of vibration and
  position sense
• ataxia
• positive Romberg test
• weakness, spasticity
• paraplegia
• hyperreflexia
• positive Babinski reflex

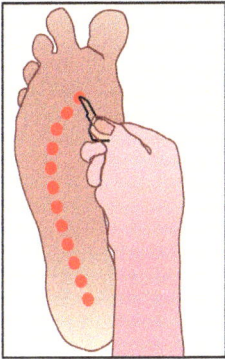

tachycardia
congestive heart failure

palpable spleen tip

pain
nausea
vomitting

bladder distension

Babinski reflex

sensorimotor peripheral
neuropathy

*Why might this patient
develop jaundice?*

Polycythemia Vera

Ocular

- conjunctival injection
- retinal vessel engorgement
- retinal artery occlusion
- visual disturbance

Nasal

- epistaxis

Oral

- bleeding gums

Integumentary

- plethoric face
- erythromelalgia
  - red, warm, painful hands
- pruritis
- skin excoriations

Arterial

- hypertension

Abdominal

- hepatomegaly
- splenomegaly
- pain and distension
  - mesenteric thrombosis
  - Budd-Chiari syndrome

Rheumatologic

- gout tophi

Neurologic

- headache
- dizziness
- vertigo
- stroke

Hematologic

- thromboses and thromboembolism
- bleeding

Polycythmia Vera

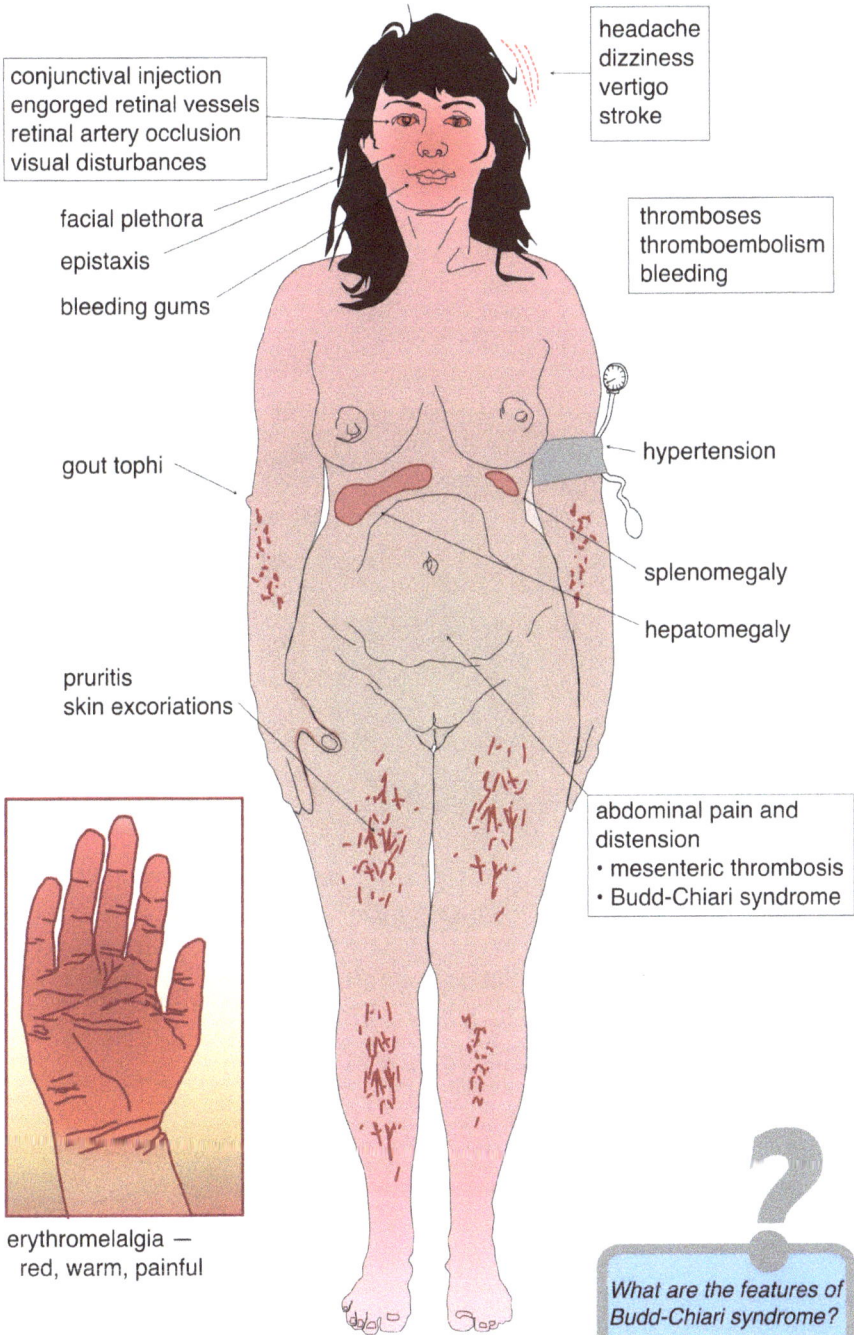

conjunctival injection
engorged retinal vessels
retinal artery occlusion
visual disturbances

headache
dizziness
vertigo
stroke

facial plethora

epistaxis

bleeding gums

thromboses
thromboembolism
bleeding

gout tophi

hypertension

splenomegaly

hepatomegaly

pruritis
skin excoriations

abdominal pain and
distension
• mesenteric thrombosis
• Budd-Chiari syndrome

erythromelalgia —
red, warm, painful

What are the features of
Budd-Chiari syndrome?

General

- weight loss
- edema

Ocular

- periorbital ecchymoses ("racoon eyes")

Oropharyngeal

- macroglossia
- hoarseness
- obstructive sleep apnea

Lymphatic

- lymphadenopathy

Integumentary

- alopecia – diffuse or patchy
- waxy papules, nodules, plaques
- purpura
- petechiae
- ecchymoses
- hypohidrosis
- brittle, crumbling nails

Cardiac

- arrhythmia
- congestive heart failure

Arterial

- postural hypotension

Pulmonary

- pleural effusion

Abdominal

- hepatomegaly
- splenomegaly
- intestinal pseudo-obstruction
- gastrointestinal hemorrhage

Musculoskeletal

- enlarged shoulder ("shoulder pad" sign)
- muscle weakness – pseudomyopathy

Neurologic

- symmetric distal neuropathy
- carpal tunnel syndrome
- autonomic neuropathies

Primary Systemic Amyloidosis

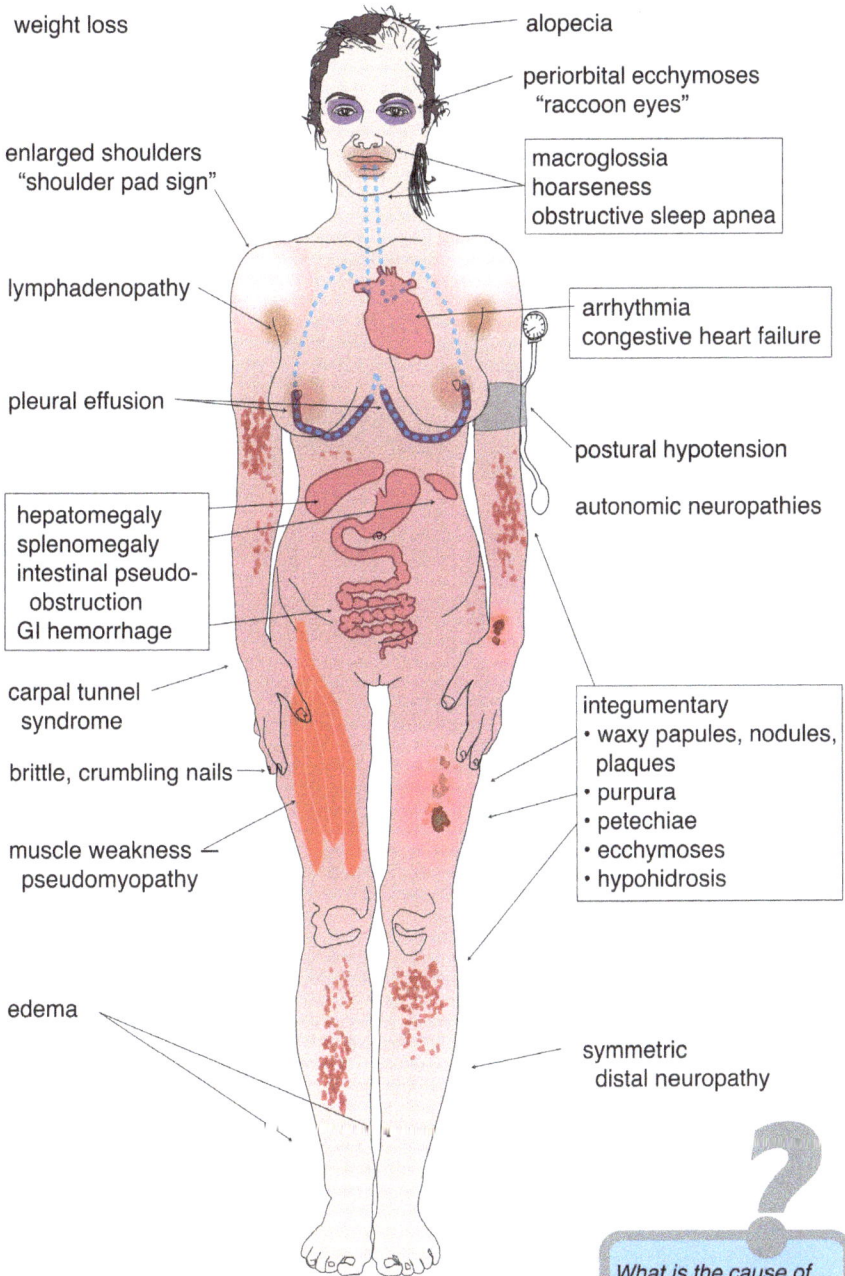

weight loss

alopecia

periorbital ecchymoses
"raccoon eyes"

enlarged shoulders
"shoulder pad sign"

macroglossia
hoarseness
obstructive sleep apnea

lymphadenopathy

arrhythmia
congestive heart failure

pleural effusion

postural hypotension

autonomic neuropathies

hepatomegaly
splenomegaly
intestinal pseudo-
obstruction
GI hemorrhage

carpal tunnel
syndrome

integumentary
• waxy papules, nodules,
  plaques
• purpura
• petechiae
• ecchymoses
• hypohidrosis

brittle, crumbling nails

muscle weakness
pseudomyopathy

edema

symmetric
distal neuropathy

?

*What is the cause of
the "shoulder pad sign"?*

Thrombotic Thrombocytopenic Purpura (TTP)

General

- fever
- fatigue
- pallor
- jaundice

Integumentary

- petechiae
- ecchymoses

Cardiac

- acute myocardial infarction
- arrythmia
- congestive heart failure
- cardiogenic shock

Abdominal

- vomiting
- diarrhea

Renal

- dark urine
- oligoanuria

Rheumatologic

- arthralgia
- myalgia
- back pain

Neurologic

- headache
- mental changes
- focal signs
- seizures
- coma

The TTP pentad:

- neurologic dysfunction
- renal insufficiency
- fever
- thrombocytopenia
- anemia

Thrombotic Thrombocytopenic Purpura (TTP)

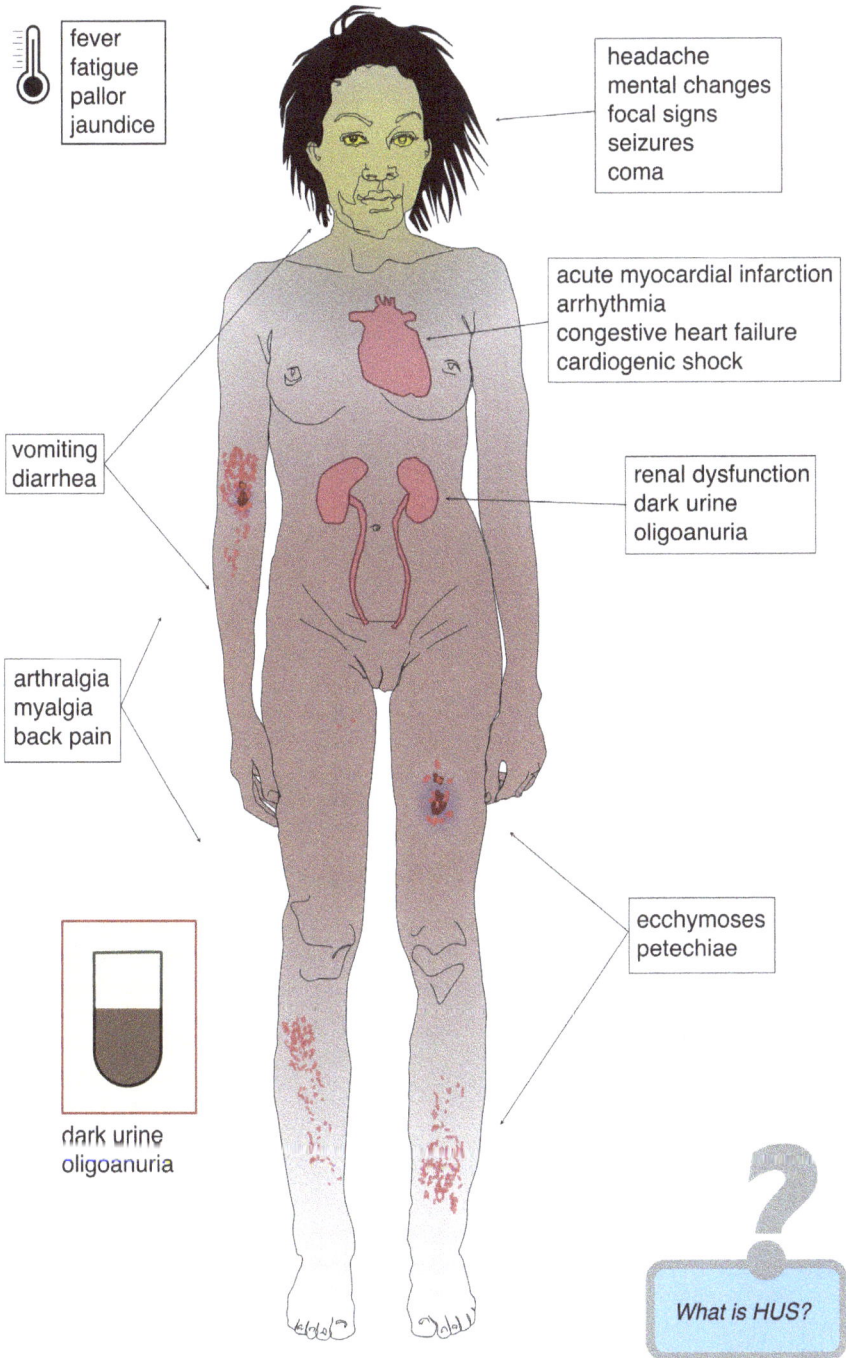

fever
fatigue
pallor
jaundice

headache
mental changes
focal signs
seizures
coma

acute myocardial infarction
arrhythmia
congestive heart failure
cardiogenic shock

vomiting
diarrhea

renal dysfunction
dark urine
oligoanuria

arthralgia
myalgia
back pain

ecchymoses
petechiae

dark urine
oligoanuria

What is HUS?

INFECTIOUS DISEASE

See also

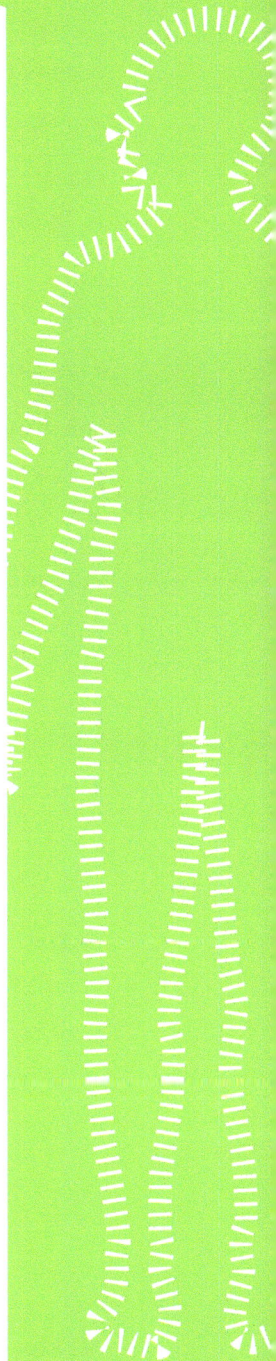

COVID-19

COVID-19 (coronavirus disease 2019) is caused by the SARS-CoV-2 virus.

General
- fever
- fatigue (profound)

Ocular
- conjunctivitis ("pink eye")

Nasal
- anosmia (loss of smell)
- nasal congestion, discharge

Oropharyngeal
- sore throat, inflammation
- ageusia (loss of taste)

Integumentary
- COVID toes (pseudo-chilblains) – swollen, red or purple toes
- vesicular eruptions (chicken pox–like)
- maculopapular rashes
- urticaria
- livedo reticularis

Cardiac
- arrhythmia
- myocarditis
- myocardial infarction
- septic shock

Pulmonary
- cough (debilitating)
- dyspnea
- pneumonia signs
- pulmonary embolism
- acute respiratory distress syndrome (ARDS)

Abdominal
- vomiting
- diarrhea

Renal
- acute kidney injury – volume overload

Rheumatologic
- myopathy
- myalgia

Neurologic
- headache, dizziness, confusion
- stroke signs
- polyneuropathy

Hematologic
- thromboses and embolisms – arterial and venous
  - brain, lungs, kidneys, extremities

COVID-19

fever
fatigue

headache, dizziness, confusion
stroke signs

sore throat
loss of taste

conjunctivitis
"pink eye"

loss of smell
nasal congestion

cough
dyspnea
pneumonia
pulmonary embolism
ARDS

arrhythmia
myocarditis
septic shock
myocardial infarction

vomiting
diarrhea

arterial and venous
thromboses and
embolisms
• brain
• lungs
• kidneys
• extremities

myopathy
myalgia

acute kidney injury
volume overload

integumentary
• COVID toes
• vesicular eruptions
• maculopapular rashes
• urticaria
• livedo reticularis

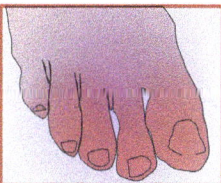

polyneuropathy

COVID toes

*What do the acronyms,
SARS and MERS,
mean?*

HIV/AIDS

Clinical signs of HIV/AIDS are predominantly those of opportunistic infections and malignancies, occurring singly or as multiple comorbidities. All body systems may be involved. The following are partial lists of signs.

General
- fever
- muscle wasting
- lipodystrophy

Ocular
- chorioretinitis
- retinal detachment
- keratoconjunctivitis

Oral
- candidiasis
- hairy leukoplakia
- necrotizing ulcerations
- gingivitis
- periodontitis
- pharyngitis

Lymphatic
- lymphadenopathy

Integumentary
- Kaposi sarcoma
- herpes zoster
- squamous cell carcinoma
- molluscum contagiosum
- perianal disease

Pulmonary
- sinusitis
- cough
- tachypnea
- pulmonary rales
- pneumonia

Cardiac
- myocarditis
- pericarditis
- coronary artery disease

Gastrointestinal
- esophagitis
- hepatosplenomegaly
- chronic diarrhea

Rheumatologic
- myositis

Neurologic
- dementia complex
- headache
- meningitis
- encephalitis
- myelopathy
- peripheral neuropathy

HIV/AIDS

Most signs are due to opportunistic infections and malignancies

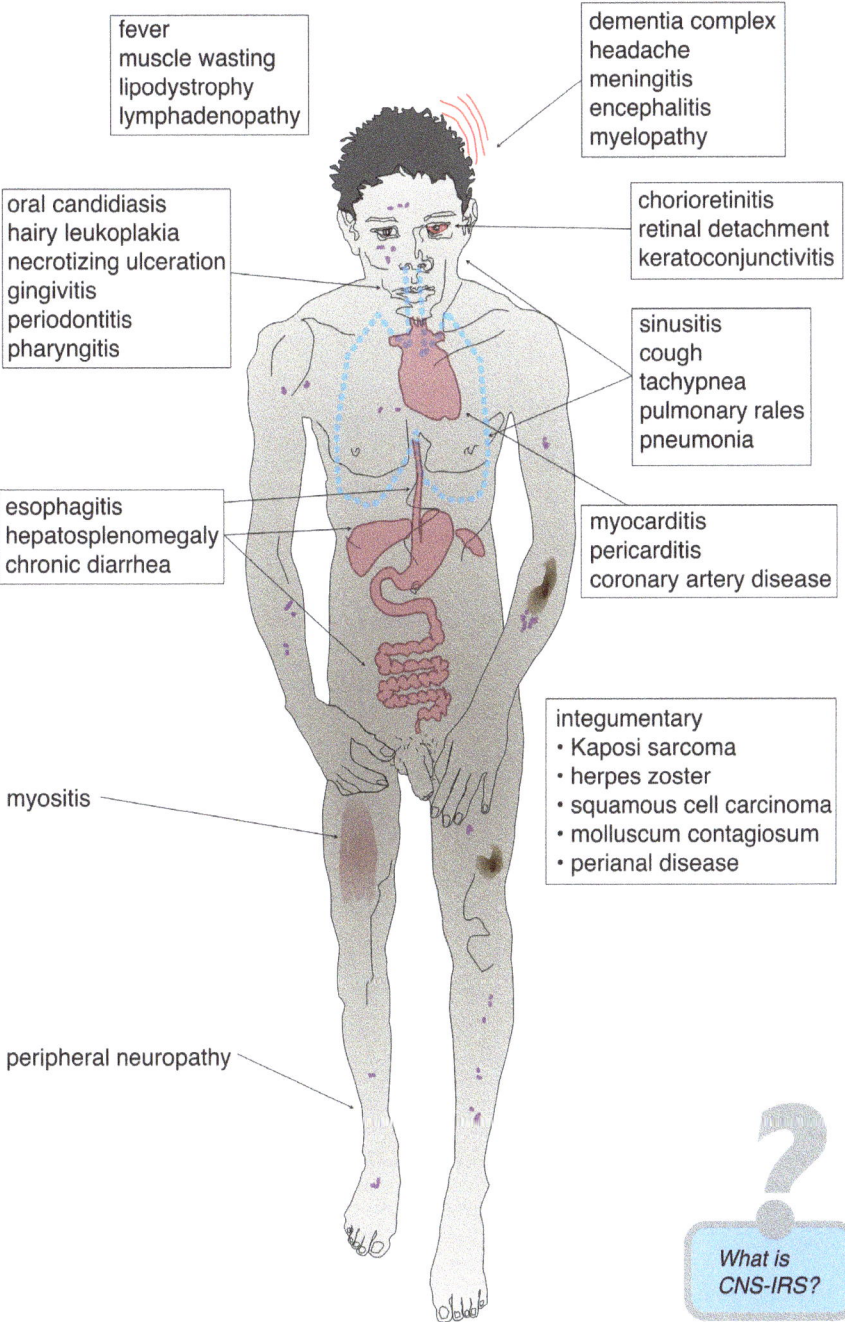

fever
muscle wasting
lipodystrophy
lymphadenopathy

dementia complex
headache
meningitis
encephalitis
myelopathy

oral candidiasis
hairy leukoplakia
necrotizing ulceration
gingivitis
periodontitis
pharyngitis

chorioretinitis
retinal detachment
keratoconjunctivitis

sinusitis
cough
tachypnea
pulmonary rales
pneumonia

esophagitis
hepatosplenomegaly
chronic diarrhea

myocarditis
pericarditis
coronary artery disease

integumentary
• Kaposi sarcoma
• herpes zoster
• squamous cell carcinoma
• molluscum contagiosum
• perianal disease

myositis

peripheral neuropathy

What is
CNS-IRS?

Lyme Disease

Clinical signs occur in stages, with some overlap.

EARLY LOCALIZED

General

- low-grade fever
- lymphadenopathy

Cutaneous

- erythema migrans
- macules or papules – >5 cm, single or multiple
- bull's-eye rash (infrequent)

EARLY DISSEMINATED

Cardiac

- atrioventricular (AV) block – bradycardia
- myocarditis, S3 gallop
- congestive heart failure

Neurologic

- cranial nerve deficits, bilateral facial nerve palsy
- meningismus
- focal weakness
- ataxia

LATE PERSISTENT

Musculoskeletal

- large joint effusions, monoarticular or polyarticular
- myositis

Neurologic

- early neurologic deficits persist
- cognitive deficits
- peripheral neuropathies

Lyme Disease

low-grade fever*

lymphadenopathy*

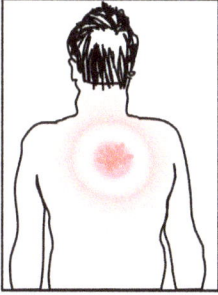

"bull's-eye" rash*

erythema migrans*
macules*
papules*

myositis***
large joint effusions***

peripheral
  neuropathies***

cranial nerve deficits**
bilateral facial nerve palsy**
cognitive deficit***
meningismus**

AV block — bradycardia**
myocarditis, S3 gallop**
congestive heart failure**

ataxia**
focal weakness**

*   early localized
**   early disseminated
*** late persistent

*How did Lyme
disease get named?*

Measles (Rubeola)

General
- fever

Ocular
- conjunctivitis (red, watery eyes)

Nasal
- coryza (watery nose)

Oral
- Koplik spots on buccal mucosa (prodromal) – opposite first and second molar; white "grains of sand" on a red base

Integumentary
- maculopapular erythematous rash – blanching; commencing on face, spreading down body, including palms and soles; coalescent
- petechiae (occasional)

Pulmonary
- cough
- measles pneumonia, or secondary bacterial pneumonia (complication)
- pleural effusion (may be sterile)

Neurologic
- encephalitis (complication)

Remember the 3 C's:
- conjunctivitis
- coryza
- cough

Measles (Rubeola)

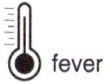

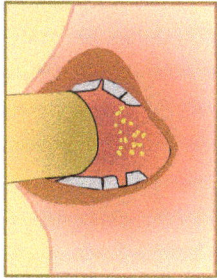

fever

encephalitis

conjunctivitis
(red, watery eyes)

coryza (watery nose)

spreading
maculopapular
erythematous rash
↓
head
↓
body
↓
palms
soles

Koplik spots —
"white grains of sand
on a red base"

cough
measles pneumonia
pleural effusion

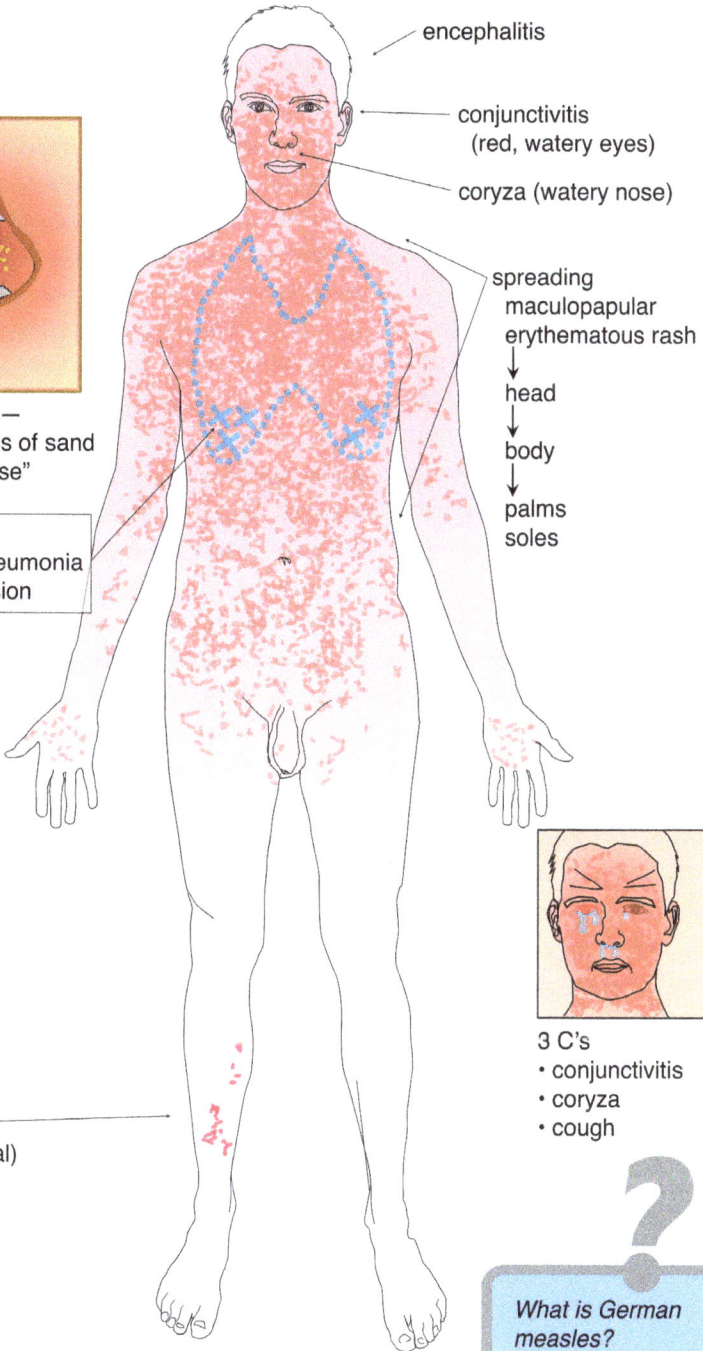

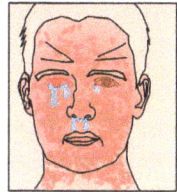

3 C's
• conjunctivitis
• coryza
• cough

petechiae
(occasional)

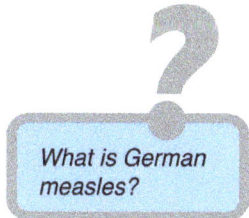

*What is German
measles?*

Meningococcal Meningitis

General

- fever

Intregumentary

- petechiae
- extensive rash
    - hemorrhagic
    - microthrombotic

Abdominal

- vomiting

Neurologic

- headache
- irritability
- altered mental state
- convulsions
- cranial nerve deficits – CN 6, 7, 8
- neck stiffness
    - Kernig sign: difficulty in extending the knee while hip is flexed
    - Brudzinski sign: flexion of the neck causes knee flexion

---

Waterhouse-Friderichsen syndrome:

- circulatory collapse
- organ failure

Classic triad of meningitis:

- fever
- neck stiffness
- altered mental state

Meningococcal Meningitis

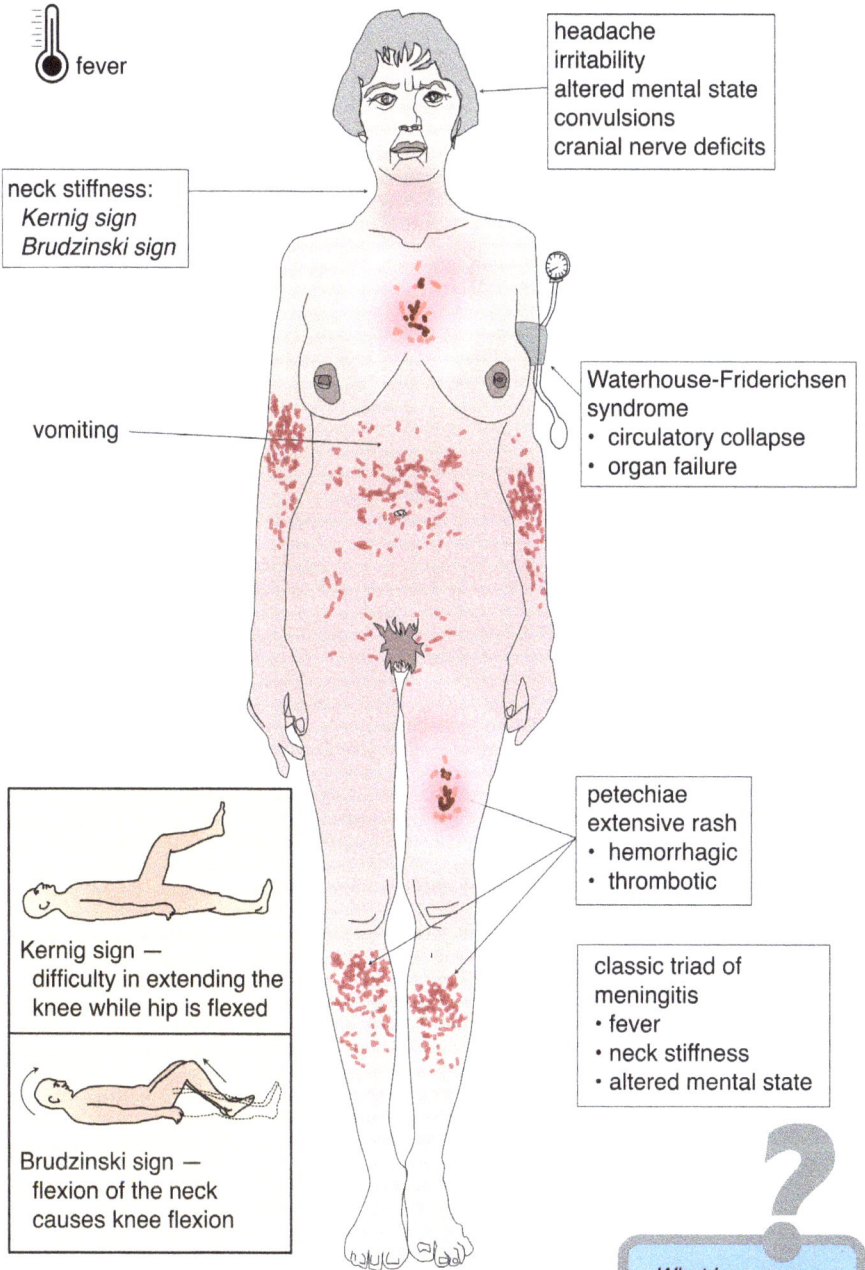

fever

headache
irritability
altered mental state
convulsions
cranial nerve deficits

neck stiffness:
Kernig sign
Brudzinski sign

Waterhouse-Friderichsen
syndrome
• circulatory collapse
• organ failure

vomiting

petechiae
extensive rash
• hemorrhagic
• thrombotic

Kernig sign —
difficulty in extending the
knee while hip is flexed

classic triad of
meningitis
• fever
• neck stiffness
• altered mental state

Brudzinski sign —
flexion of the neck
causes knee flexion

*What is purpura
fulminans?*

Tuberculosis – Pulmonary and Disseminated

General

- weight loss
- fever and sweats

Ocular

- chorioretinitis

Lymphatic

- lymphadenitis – cervical and supraclavicular

Integumentary

- scrofuloderma (especially on the neck) – papules, plaques, nodules, ulcers, sinuses
- papulonecrotic lesions on extensor surfaces
- hyperpigmentation
- lupus vulgaris – reddish-brown "apple jelly nodules"

Cardiac

- pericarditis – effusion, tamponade, constrictive

Pulmonary

- cough and hemoptysis
- consolidation and abscess cavitation (upper lobes)

Abdominal

- peritonitis
- ascites
- diarrhea

Musculoskeletal

- monoarthritis
- Pott spine: vertebral osteitis, deformity, paraplegia

Renal

- renal mass

Genitourinary

- scrotal mass, orchitis, epididymitis
- pelvic inflammatory disease

Neurologic

- headache
- meningeal signs
- confusion
- coma

Tuberculosis
Pulmonary and Disseminated

weight loss
fever and sweats

headache
meningeal signs
confusion, coma

chorioretinitis

lymphadenitis

cough, hemoptysis
consolidation
abscess cavitation

pericarditis
• effusion
• tamponade
• constrictive

renal mass

peritonitis
ascites
diarrhea

integumentary
• scrofuloderma
• papulonecrotic
• hyperpigmentation
• lupus vulgaris

pelvic inflammatory
disease (female)

scrotal mass
orchitis
epididymitis

monoarthritis

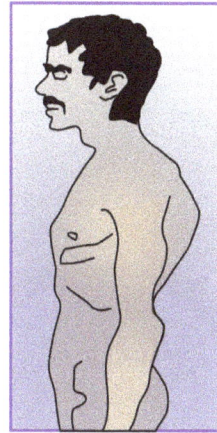

Pott spine
• vertebral osteitis
• deformity
• paraplegia

*Why was tuberculosis
called "consumption"?*

NEPHROLOGY

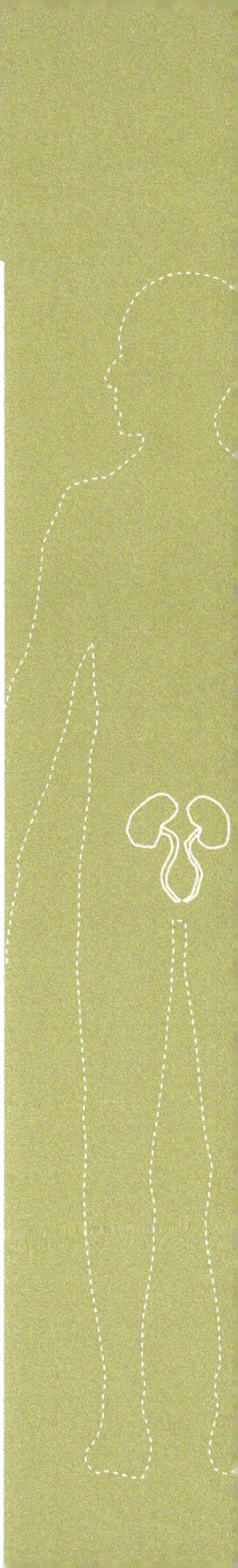

Ocular

- retinal artery occlusion

Cardiac

- valvular regurgitation
  - mitral valve prolapse
  - aortic regurgitation
- angina
- myocardial infarction

Arterial

- hypertension
- aortic aneurysm – dissection

Abdominal

- bilateral enlarged kidneys, bimanually ballotable
- cystic hepatomegaly – jaundice (bile duct compression)
- abdominal pain and tenderness, suggesting
  - cyst expansion
  - cyst hemorrhage
  - infection
  - nephrolithiasis
  - tumor
  - diverticulitis

Urinary

- hematuria

Neurologic

- stroke (intracranial bleed)

Autosomal Dominant Polycystic Kidney Disease (ADPKD)

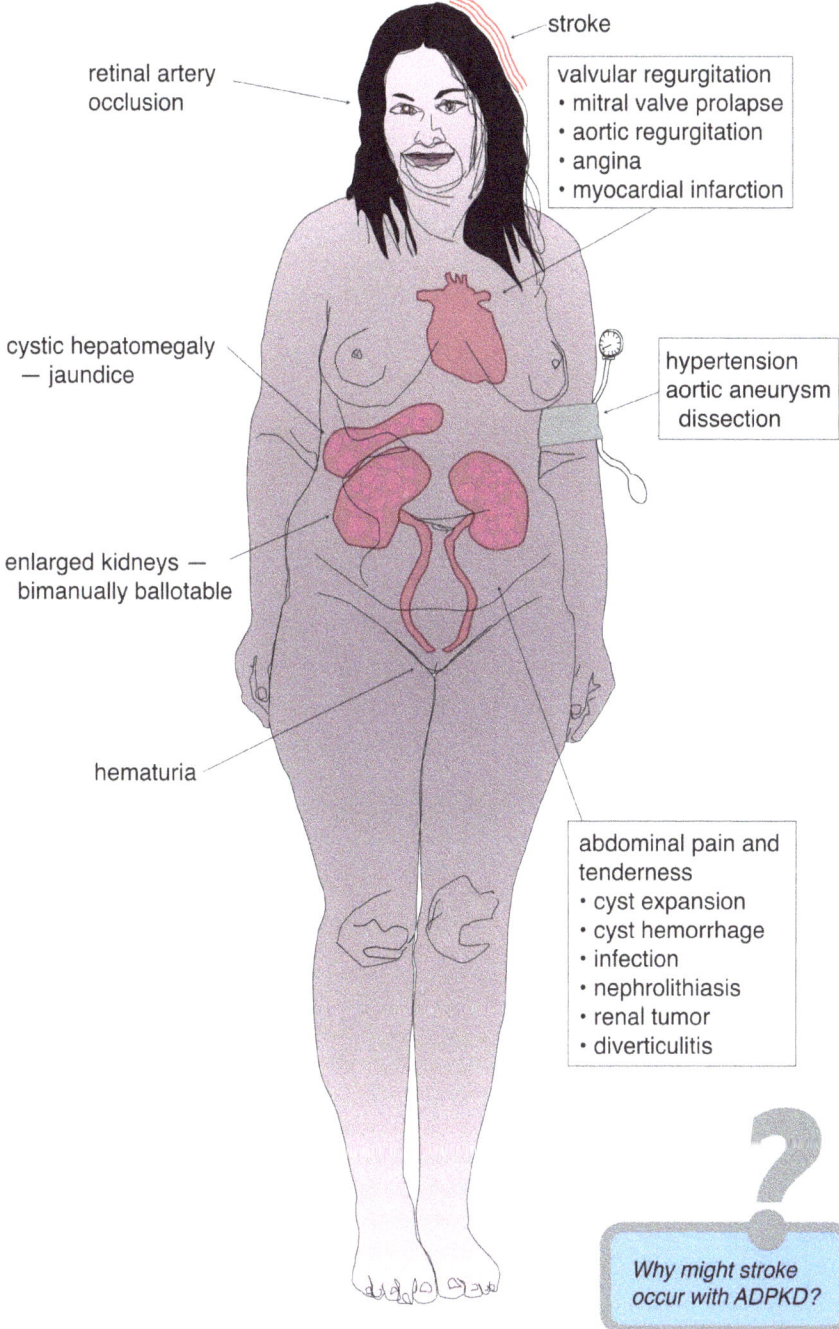

stroke

retinal artery occlusion

valvular regurgitation
- mitral valve prolapse
- aortic regurgitation
- angina
- myocardial infarction

cystic hepatomegaly — jaundice

hypertension
aortic aneurysm
dissection

enlarged kidneys — bimanually ballotable

hematuria

abdominal pain and tenderness
- cyst expansion
- cyst hemorrhage
- infection
- nephrolithiasis
- renal tumor
- diverticulitis

?

Why might stroke occur with ADPKD?

General

- fatigue
- sallow complexion
- malnutrition
- uremic fetor

Ocular

- red eye (calcium deposits)

Oral

- xerostomia
- periodontitis
- gingival hyperplasia
- bleeding gums

Integumentary

- bullous dermatoses
- xerosis, scratching
- calciphylaxis
- nephrogenic systemic fibrosis
- ecchymoses
- uremic frost

Cardiac

- valvular stenosis (calcification)
- pericardial rub
- pericardial effusion
- congestive heart failure (CHF)
- peripheral edema

Arterial

- hypertension

Pulmonary

- Kussmaul breathing
- pleural rub
- pulmonary edema

Gastrointestinal

- vomiting, diarrhea
- gastrointestinal bleeding

Musculoskeletal

- muscle weakness, cramps
- bone pain, fractures

Neurologic

- asterixis (uremic flap)
- uremic encephalopathy

Plus, signs of the underlying condition

Chronic Kidney Failure and Uremia

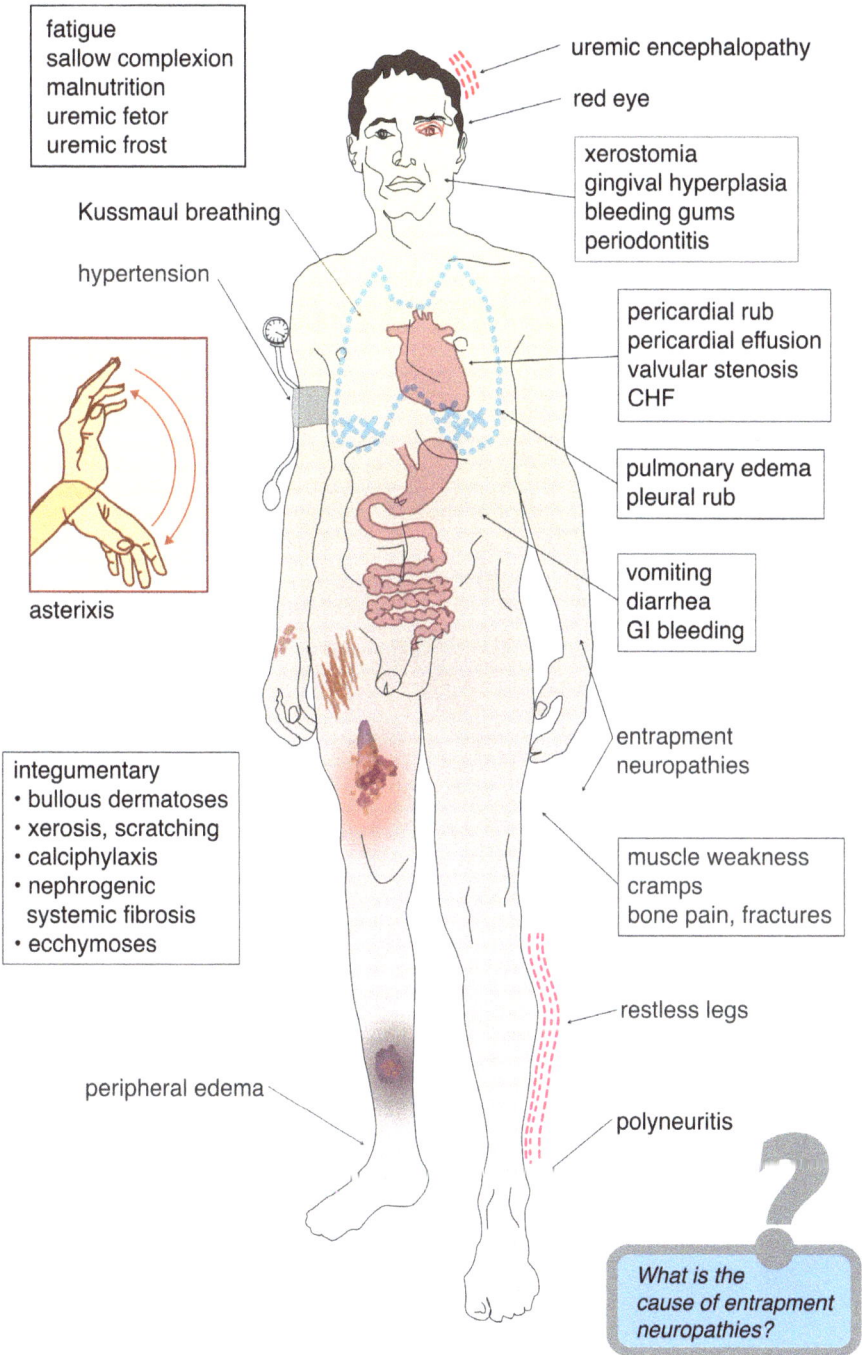

fatigue
sallow complexion
malnutrition
uremic fetor
uremic frost

uremic encephalopathy

red eye

xerostomia
gingival hyperplasia
bleeding gums
periodontitis

Kussmaul breathing

hypertension

pericardial rub
pericardial effusion
valvular stenosis
CHF

pulmonary edema
pleural rub

vomiting
diarrhea
GI bleeding

asterixis

entrapment
neuropathies

muscle weakness
cramps
bone pain, fractures

integumentary
• bullous dermatoses
• xerosis, scratching
• calciphylaxis
• nephrogenic
  systemic fibrosis
• ecchymoses

restless legs

peripheral edema

polyneuritis

*What is the
cause of entrapment
neuropathies?*

Minimal Change Disease (MCD)

General

- weight gain (sudden)
- periorbital edema
- xanthelasma and xanthomas
- peripheral edema
- anasarca
- white nails, Muehrcke lines

Arterial

- normal blood pressure

Venous

- venous thrombosis (peripheral)

Pulmonary

- pleural effusion
- pulmonary embolism

Abdominal

- ascites
- peritonitis (bacterial)
- pancreatitis

Urinary

- frothy urine

Potential associated conditions:
- Hodgkin lymphoma: lymphadenopathy, splenomegaly
- mycosis fungoides: red, scaly skin rash, small papules

Minimal Change Disease (MCD)

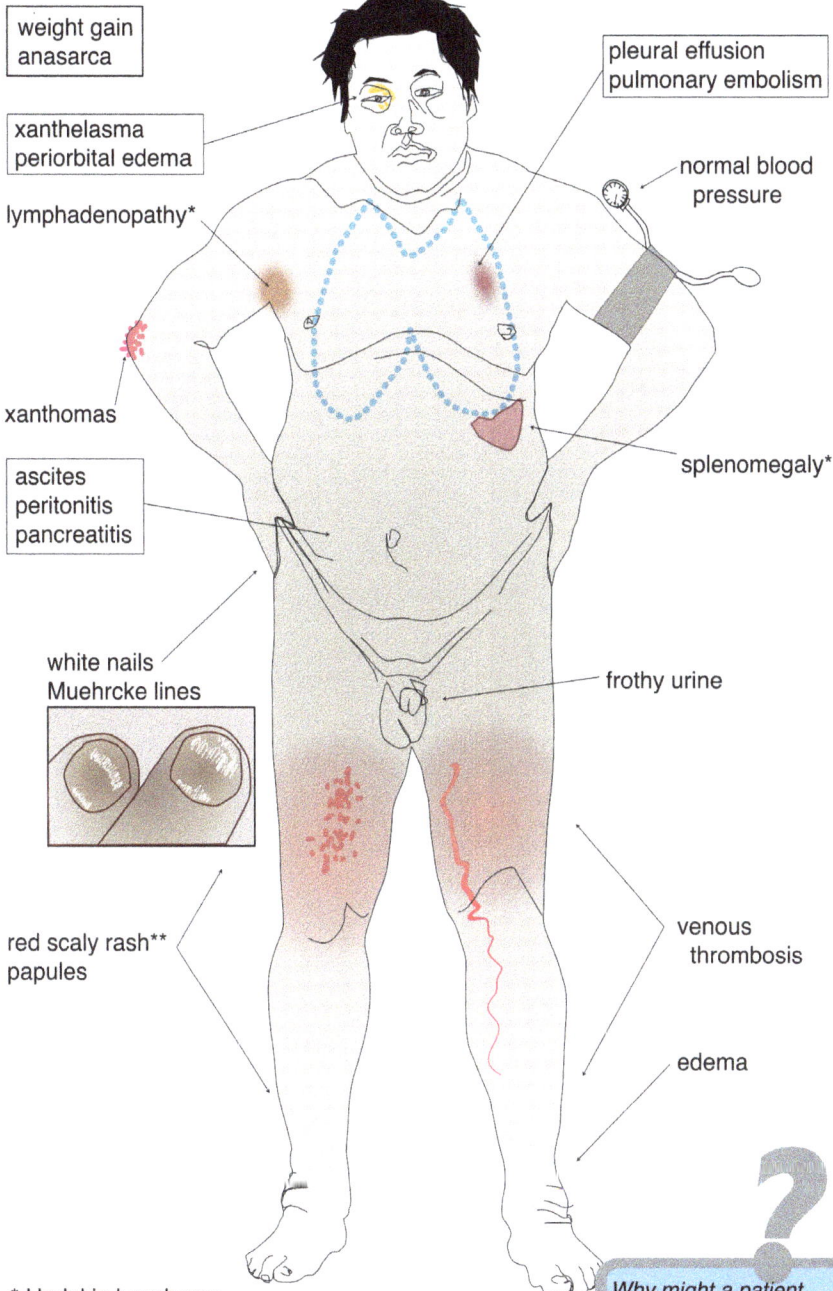

weight gain
anasarca

pleural effusion
pulmonary embolism

xanthelasma
periorbital edema

normal blood
pressure

lymphadenopathy*

xanthomas

splenomegaly*

ascites
peritonitis
pancreatitis

white nails
Muehrcke lines

frothy urine

red scaly rash**
papules

venous
thrombosis

edema

* Hodgkin lymphoma
**mycosis fungoides

*Why might a patient
with nephrotic syndrome
develop peritonitis?*

Glomerulonephritis – Post-Streptococcal Glomerulonephritis

General

- lethargy
- fever
- edema
  - periorbital
  - peripheral
  - anasarca

Cardiac

- left ventricular dysfunction

Arterial

- hypertension

Urinary

- hematuria with cola-colored urine
- frothy urine

Complicated acute PSGN:
- pallor
- hypertensive encephalopathy
- seizures
- hypoxic respiratory failure

Glomerulonephritis
Post-Streptococcal Glomerulonephritis (PSGN)

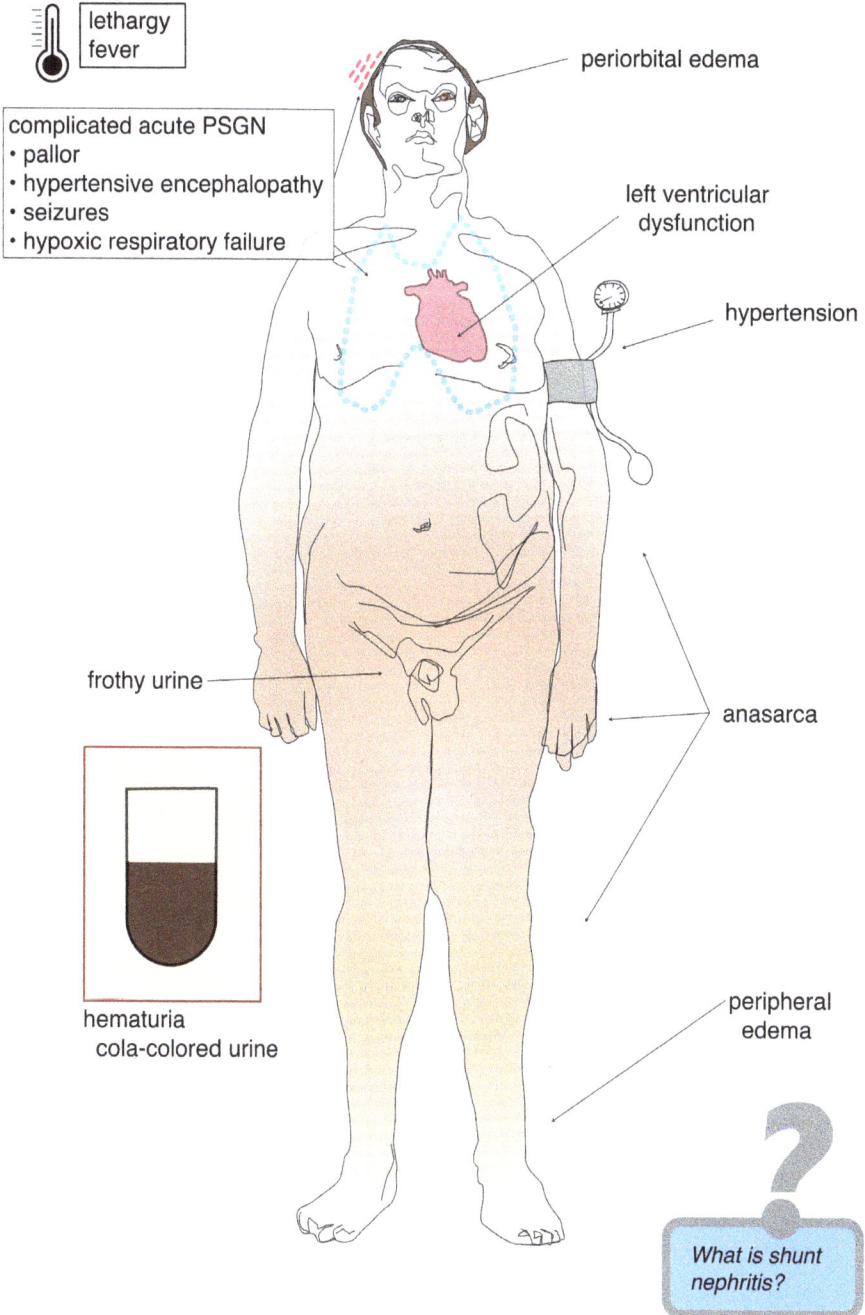

lethargy
fever

complicated acute PSGN
• pallor
• hypertensive encephalopathy
• seizures
• hypoxic respiratory failure

periorbital edema

left ventricular
dysfunction

hypertension

frothy urine

anasarca

hematuria
cola-colored urine

peripheral
edema

*What is shunt
nephritis?*

Renal Small Vessel Vasculitis

Extrarenal signs are presented for immune complex renal small vessel vasculitis and pauci-immune renal small vessel vasculitis.

Immune complex small vessel vasculitis, including the following conditions:

- anti-glomerular basement membrane (anti-GBM) disease (Goodpasture disease)
- cryoglobulinemic vasculitis
- IgA vasculitis (Henoch-Schönlein purpura)
- hypocomplementemic urticarial vasculitis (anti-C1q vasculitis)
- systemic lupus erythematosus (SLE)

General: fever, weight loss

Ocular: inflammation – retinal vasculitis, optic neuritis

Integumentary: butterfly rash, purpura, skin photosensitivity (with SLE), skin ulcerations

Cardiac: myocarditis, pericarditis

Pulmonary: pleuritis, pulmonary hemorrhage (for anti-GBM, the sole extrarenal sign)

Abdominal: abdominal pain, bloody stools

Urinary: hematuria

Rheumatologic: arthritis

Neurologic: headache, seizures, peripheral neuropathies, mononeuritis multiplex

Pauci-immune small vessel vasculitis, including the following conditions:

- granulomatosis with polyangiitis (GPA) (Wegener granulomatosis)
- microscopic polyangiitis (MPA)
- eosinophilic granulomatosis with polyangiitis (EGPA) (Churg-Strauss syndrome)

General: fever, weight loss

Ocular: inflammation – scleritis, uveitis

Nasal: sinusitis, rhinitis saddle nose deformity and septal perforation (not with MPA)

Integumentary: purpura, nodular skin lesions, ulcerations

Cardiac: myocarditis, heart block

Pulmonary: pulmonary hemorrhage, subglottic tracheal stenosis, asthma (EGPA)

Abdominal: abdominal pain, bloody stools

Urinary: hematuria

Rheumatologic: arthritis

Neurologic: headache, seizures, peripheral neuropathies, mononeuritis multiplex

Renal Small Vessel Vasculitis

(Extrarenal Signs)

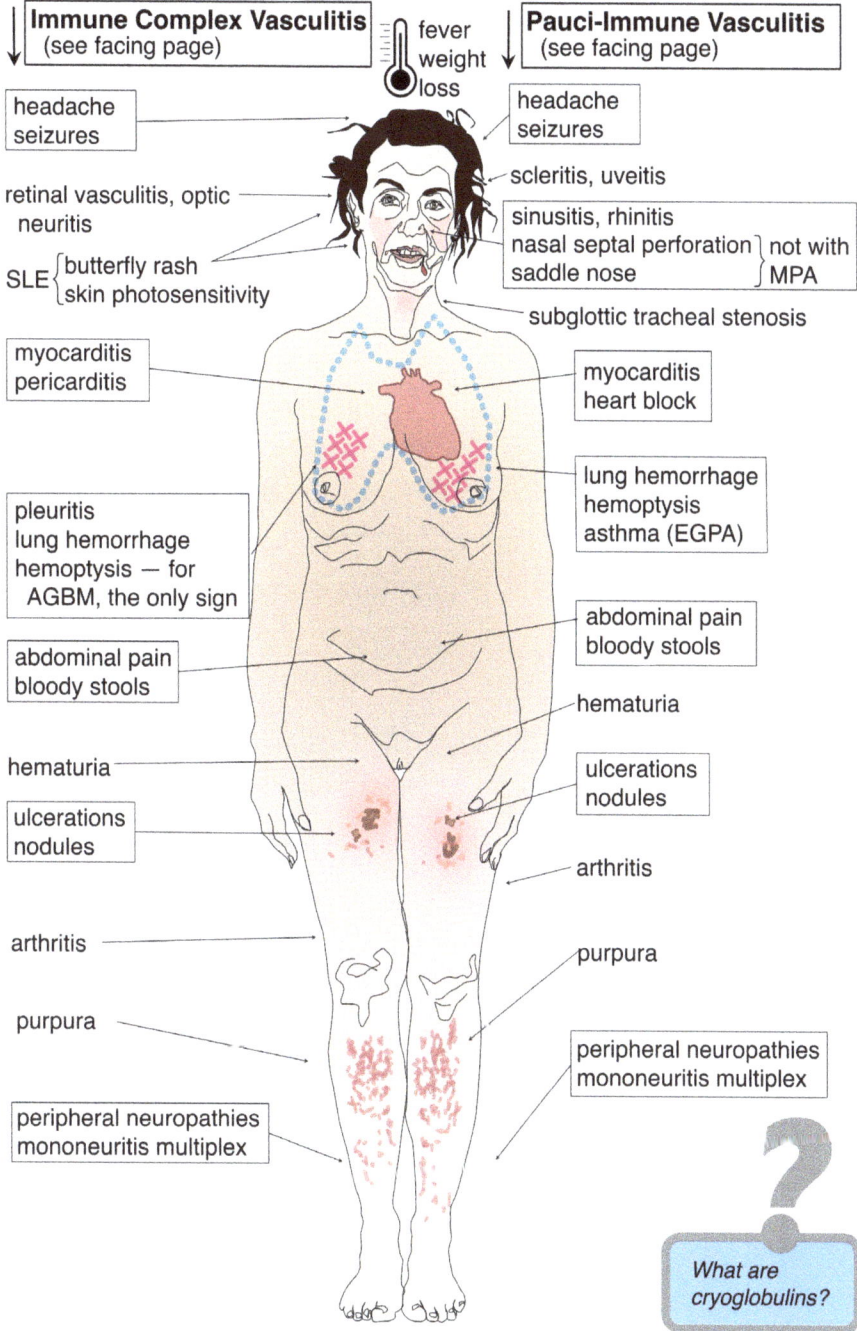

Immune Complex Vasculitis
(see facing page)

fever
weight
loss

Pauci-Immune Vasculitis
(see facing page)

headache
seizures

headache
seizures

scleritis, uveitis

retinal vasculitis, optic
neuritis

sinusitis, rhinitis
nasal septal perforation ⎫ not with
saddle nose ⎭ MPA

SLE ⎰ butterfly rash
⎱ skin photosensitivity

subglottic tracheal stenosis

myocarditis
pericarditis

myocarditis
heart block

lung hemorrhage
hemoptysis
asthma (EGPA)

pleuritis
lung hemorrhage
hemoptysis — for
  AGBM, the only sign

abdominal pain
bloody stools

abdominal pain
bloody stools

hematuria

hematuria

ulcerations
nodules

ulcerations
nodules

arthritis

arthritis

purpura

purpura

peripheral neuropathies
mononeuritis multiplex

peripheral neuropathies
mononeuritis multiplex

?

*What are
cryoglobulins?*

Screen for syndromes associated with secondary hypertension.

Hyperthyroidism

- goitre
- hyperkinetic state
- sweating
- fine tremor

Cushing Disease

- truncal obesity
- moon face
- buffalo hump
- purple striae

Acromegaly

- coarse face, broad nose
- large hands and feet

Primary Hyperaldosteronism

- muscle weakness
- muscle cramps, tetany

Pheochromocytoma

- paroxysmal hypertension
- episodic headaches
- palpitations
- diaphoresis

Obstructive Sleep Apnea

- short neck, increased circumference
- obesity
- large tongue

Coarctation of the Aorta

- hypoplastic aortic arch
- arm blood pressure >20 mmHg greater than leg
- delayed or diminished femoral pulse

Renovascular Disease

- abdominal bruits
- diffuse arteriosclerosis
- flash pulmonary edema

Renal Parenchymal Disease

- pallor
- edema
- hematuria

Drug Use

- needle track marks

Secondary Hypertension

Screen for syndromes associated with hypertension

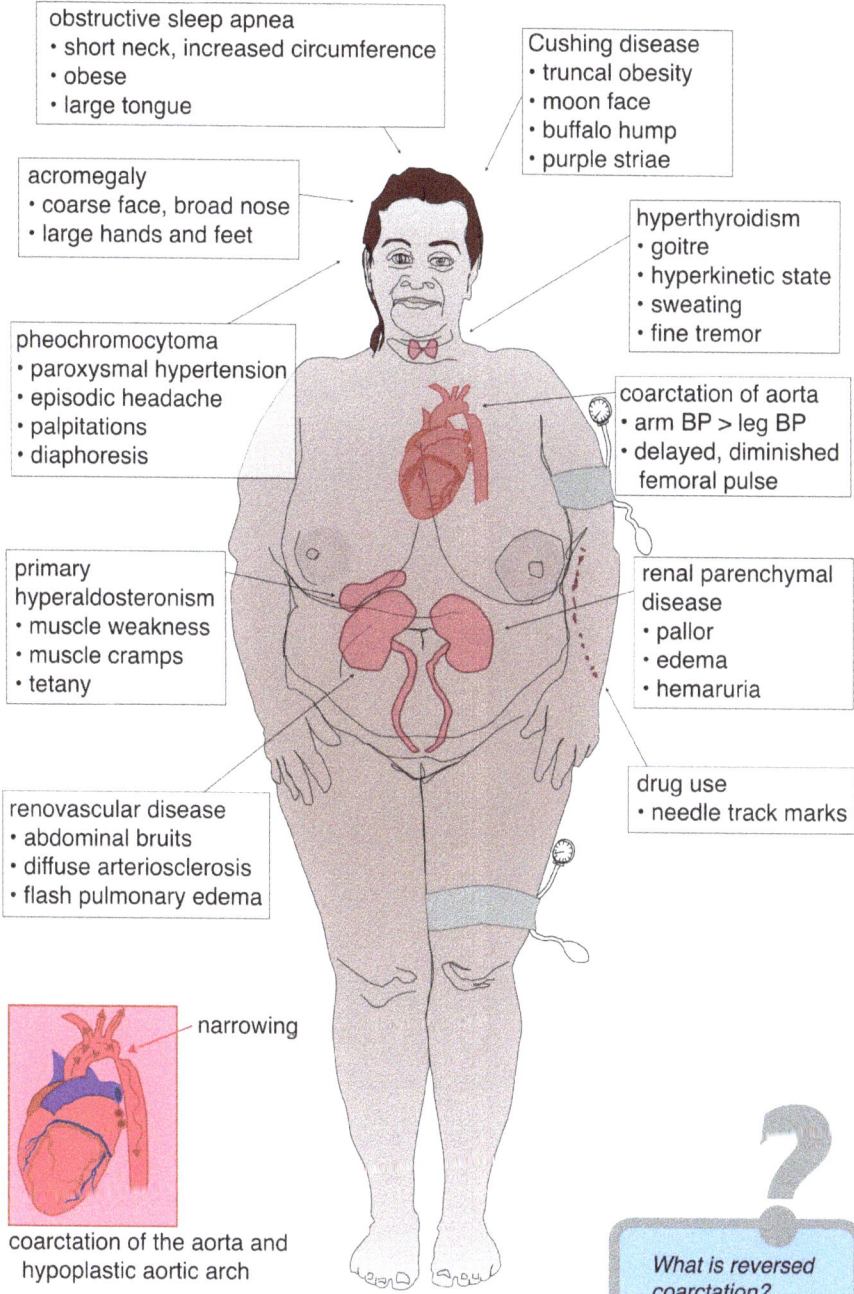

obstructive sleep apnea
• short neck, increased circumference
• obese
• large tongue

Cushing disease
• truncal obesity
• moon face
• buffalo hump
• purple striae

acromegaly
• coarse face, broad nose
• large hands and feet

hyperthyroidism
• goitre
• hyperkinetic state
• sweating
• fine tremor

pheochromocytoma
• paroxysmal hypertension
• episodic headache
• palpitations
• diaphoresis

coarctation of aorta
• arm BP > leg BP
• delayed, diminished
  femoral pulse

primary
hyperaldosteronism
• muscle weakness
• muscle cramps
• tetany

renal parenchymal
disease
• pallor
• edema
• hemaruria

drug use
• needle track marks

renovascular disease
• abdominal bruits
• diffuse arteriosclerosis
• flash pulmonary edema

narrowing

coarctation of the aorta and
hypoplastic aortic arch

What is reversed
coarctation?

NEUROLOGY

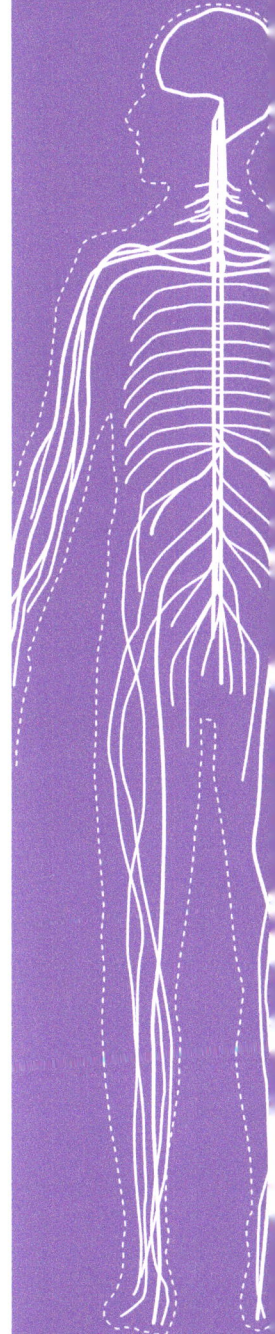

Amyotrophic Lateral Sclerosis (ALS)

ALS includes a variable combination of upper motor neuron and lower motor neuron signs. Preserved or increased reflex in a wasted extremity is a hallmark of ALS. Onset is most frequently in the extremities, then secondarily bulbar and less often pulmonary and truncal/abdominal (axial).

Limb Onset

- upper motor neuron (UMN) signs:
  - rigidity
  - impaired dexterity despite normal muscle strength
  - hyperreflexia
  - extensor plantar reflex (Babinski reflex)
- lower motor neuron (LMN) signs:
  - muscle atrophy
  - flaccidity
  - fasciculations
  - diminished reflexes
  - foot drop

Pulmonary and Truncal/Abdominal (Axial)

- dyspnea
- paradoxical chest-abdominal motion

Bulbar Onset

- upper motor neuron (UMN) signs:
  - brisk jaw jerk
  - tongue spasticity
  - palatal spasticity
  - dysarthria
  - dysphagia
  - pseudobulbar palsy
- lower motor neuron (LMN) signs:
  - wasted tongue
  - tongue fibrillation
  - low palatal elevation
  - weak facial muscles
  - weak neck muscles (dropped head syndrome)

Neuropsychiatric

- impaired executive function
- dementia
- emotional lability

Amyotrophic Lateral Sclerosis

dementia
impaired executive function
emotional lability

LMN Signs
• weak facial muscles
• wasted tongue
• tongue fibrillation
• low palate

UMN Signs
• brisk jaw jerk
• tongue spasticity
• palatal spasticity
• dysarthria
• dysphagia
• pseudobulbar palsy

dropped head
syndrome

dyspnea
paradoxical chest-
abdominal motion

LMN Signs
• atrophy
• flaccidity
• fasciculation
• diminished reflexes

UMN Signs
• rigidity
• impaired dexterity
• hyperreflexia

extensor plantar reflex
(Basinski) (UMN)

foot drop (LMN)

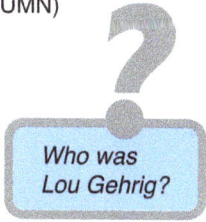

Who was
Lou Gehrig?

Guillain-Barré Syndrome

Ascending Paralysis

- symmetrical
- begins in lower extremities, moving upward
- hypotonia
- absent or diminished reflexes

Respiratory Muscle Weakness

- dyspnea
- diminished inspiratory effort

Cranial Nerve Involvement

- facial drooping
- dysphagia
- dysarthria
- oculomotor paresis

Sensory Involvement

- minimal sensory signs, but
  - numbness
  - tingling
  - pain

Autonomic Dysfunction

- cardiac arrythmias
- labile blood pressure
- temperature high or low
- paralytic ileus
- urine retention

Guillain-Barré Syndrome

temperature — high or low

facial drooping

oculomotor paresis

dysphagia

dysarthria

arrythmias

dyspnea
diminished
  inspiratory effort

labile blood
pressure

paralytic ileus

urinary retention

numbness
tingling
pain

ascending paralysis
• symmetrical
• hypotonia
• absent or diminished
  reflexes

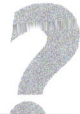

What is Miller Fisher syndrome?

Left Middle Cerebral Artery Stroke (Left Hemispheric Stroke)

Aphasia

- receptive, expressive, global

Deviation of Head and Eyes

- to the side of the infarct

Visual Defect

- right homonymous hemianopia

Apraxia

- motor apraxia

- verbal apraxia

Contralateral (Right Side) Effects

- lower facial droop

- hemiplegia, hemiparesis

- increased muscle tone +/– clasp-knife rigidity

- brisk tendon reflexes +/– ankle clonus

- Babinski reflex

- hemisensory diminished sensation

Right hemispheric stroke, conversely, affects the left side of the body:

- neglect of left side of body

- short attention span

- visual/spatial problems

Left Middle Cerebral Artery Stroke
(Left Hemispheric Stroke)

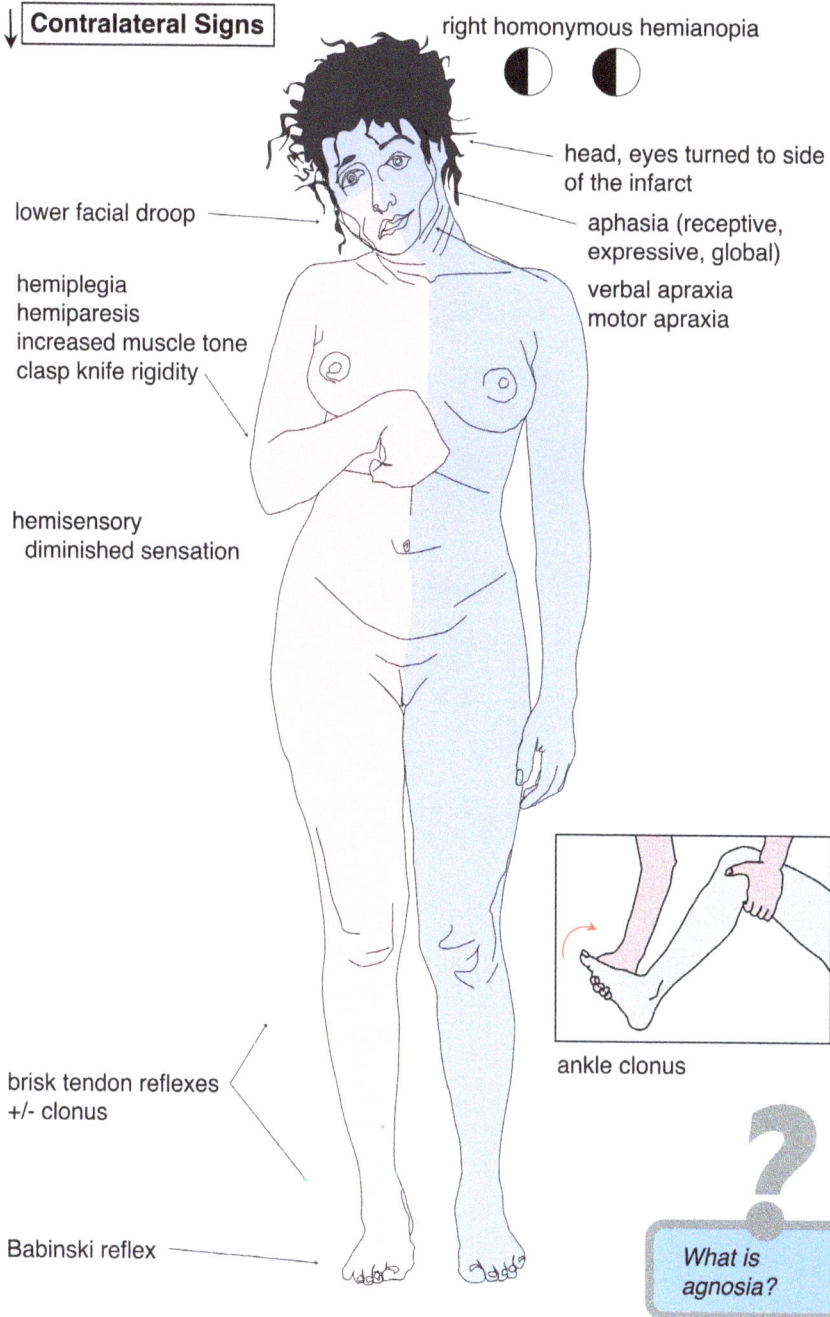

Contralateral Signs

right homonymous hemianopia

head, eyes turned to side of the infarct

lower facial droop

aphasia (receptive, expressive, global)

hemiplegia
hemiparesis
increased muscle tone
clasp knife rigidity

verbal apraxia
motor apraxia

hemisensory
 diminished sensation

ankle clonus

brisk tendon reflexes
+/- clonus

Babinski reflex

?

What is agnosia?

Parkinson Disease

Bradykinesia

- masked facies
- reduced blinking and smiling
- hypophonia (soft monotonous speech)
- sialorrhea (drooling)
- impaired swallowing
- slow, short shuffling gait and festination
- reduced arm swing
- micrographia (small handwriting)

Rigidity

- muscle rigidity
- cogwheeling

Tremor

- trembling of extremities
- pill-rolling hand tremor

Postural Instability

- stooped (simian) posture, forward tilt of trunk
- postural sway and falls

Parkinson Disease

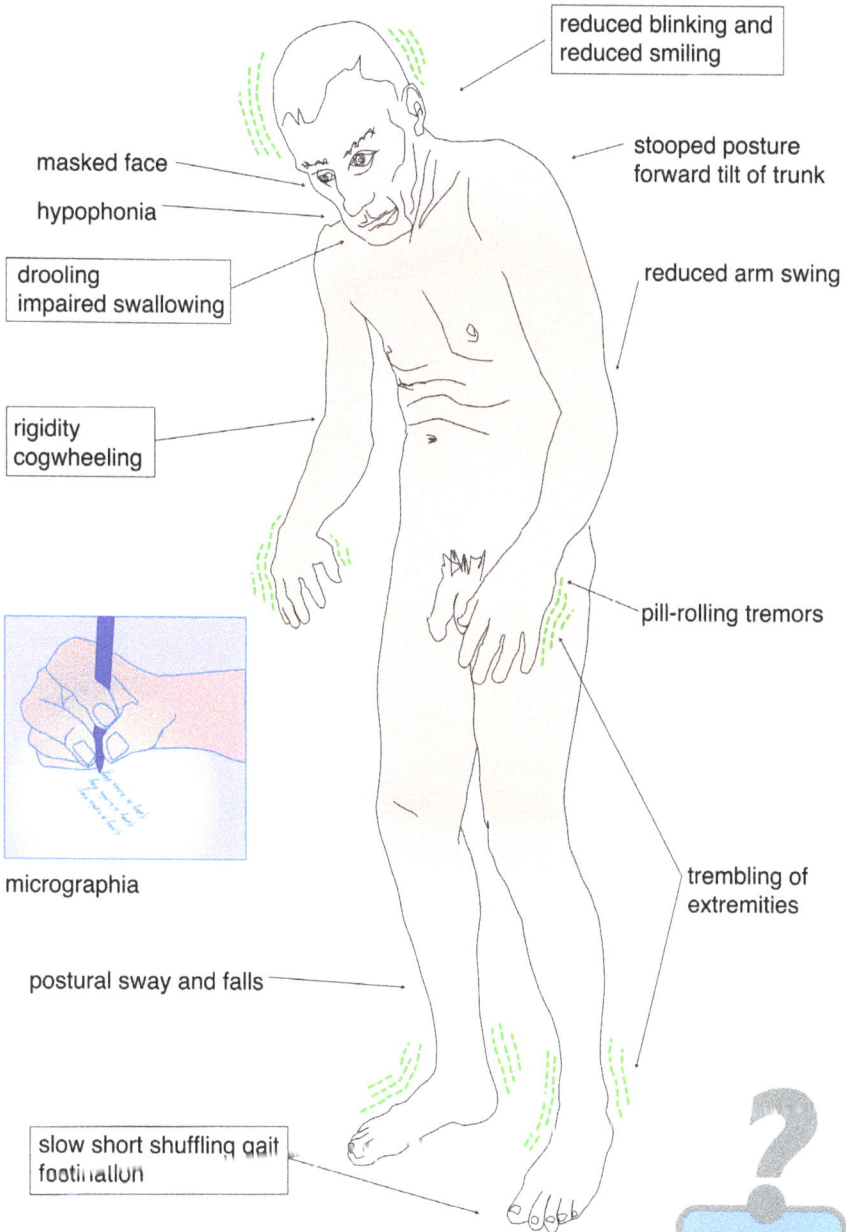

reduced blinking and reduced smiling

stooped posture forward tilt of trunk

masked face

hypophonia

reduced arm swing

drooling
impaired swallowing

rigidity
cogwheeling

pill-rolling tremors

micrographia

trembling of extremities

postural sway and falls

slow short shuffling gait
footi... ation

What is the "pull test"?

Spinal Stenosis

The clinical signs depend on whether the stenosis is located at the level of the cervical or lumbar spine.

Cervical Spinal Stenosis

- dermatomal impaired sensation
- impaired finger dexterity
- diminished reflexes
- myelopathy
  - lower extremity weakness
  - hyperreflexia
  - spasticity
  - Babinski sign
  - ataxia
  - decreased position sense
  - Romberg sign

Lumbar Spinal Stenosis

- wide gait
- decreased lordosis with forward flexion gait
- thigh pain with lumbar extension, decreased with leaning forward or sitting
- neurogenic claudication: radiating leg pain when walking
- cauda equina syndrome: bilateral leg weakness, urine retention (rare)
- positive stoop test*

Stoop test: Patient is instructed to walk with exaggerated lumbar lordosis until neurogenic claudication occurs or is worsened. The patient is then instructed to lean forward. The test is positive if symptoms are reduced.

Spinal Stenosis

Cervical Spinal Stenosis

Lumbar Spinal Stenosis

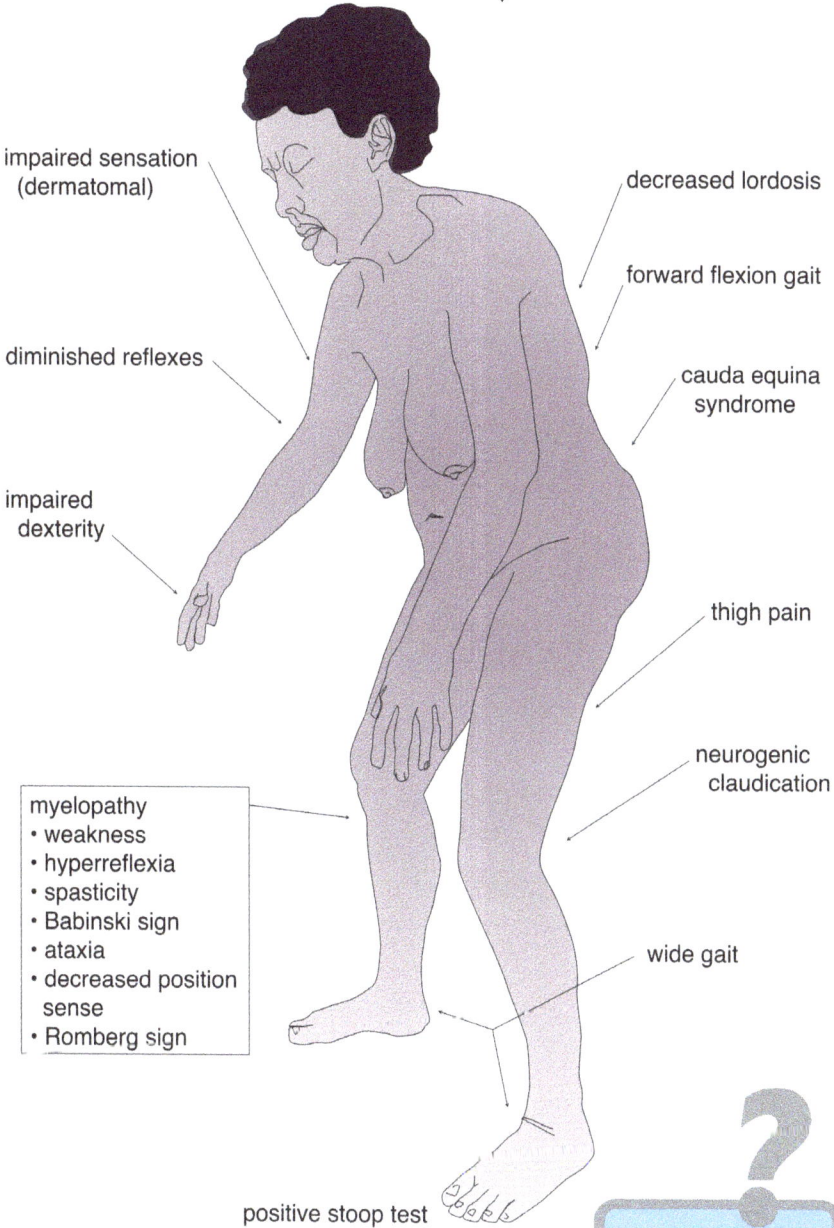

impaired sensation
(dermatomal)

diminished reflexes

impaired
dexterity

decreased lordosis

forward flexion gait

cauda equina
syndrome

thigh pain

neurogenic
claudication

myelopathy
• weakness
• hyperreflexia
• spasticity
• Babinski sign
• ataxia
• decreased position
  sense
• Romberg sign

wide gait

positive stoop test

?

*What are the causes
of spinal stenosis?*

PULMONOLOGY

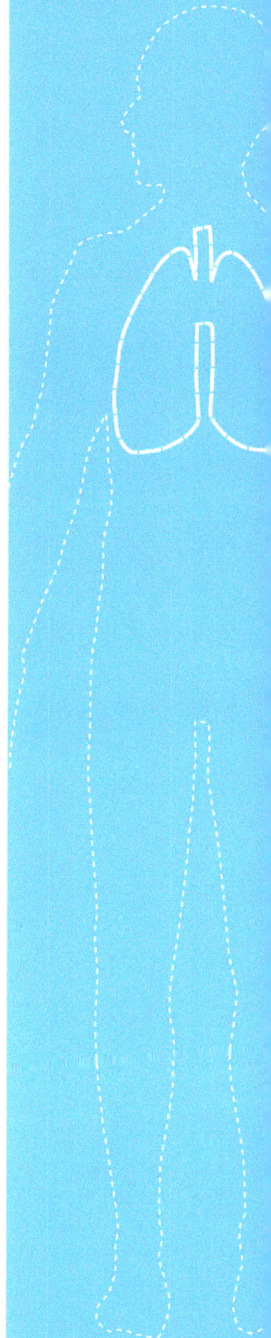

Chronic Obstructive Pulmonary Disease (COPD) – Chronic Bronchitis and Emphysema

Chronic Bronchitis (Blue Bloater)

- may be obese
- cyanosis
- plethora (polycythemia)
- pulmonary signs:
  - cough and expectoration, often mucopurulent
  - tachypnea
  - coarse rhonchi and wheezes
- cardiac signs:
  - loud P2, pulmonary hypertension
  - elevated jugular venous pressure (JVP)
  - cor pulmonale
  - peripheral edema

Emphysema (Pink Puffer)

- may be thin with muscle wasting
- pulmonary signs:
  - little or no cough
  - pursed lips during expiration
  - hyperventilation
  - hyperinflated, barrel chest
  - hyperresonance
  - prolonged expiration
  - diminished breath sounds
  - expiratory wheezing
  - coarse inspiratory crackles
- cardiac sign:
  - distant heart sounds

Chronic bronchitis and emphysema often occur in combination:

- tachypnea and respiratory distress with simple activities (when severe)
- active use of accessory respiratory muscles
- paradoxical indrawing of lower intercostal areas (Hoover sign)

Chronic Obstructive Pulmonary Disease (COPD)

Chronic Bronchitis (Blue Bloater)

may be obese

cyanosis
plethora (polycythemia)

cough
expectoration
tachypnea
coarse rhonchi and
wheezes

elevated JVP
loud P2
pulmonary hypertension
cor pulmonale

use of respiratory
accessory muscles

peripheral edema

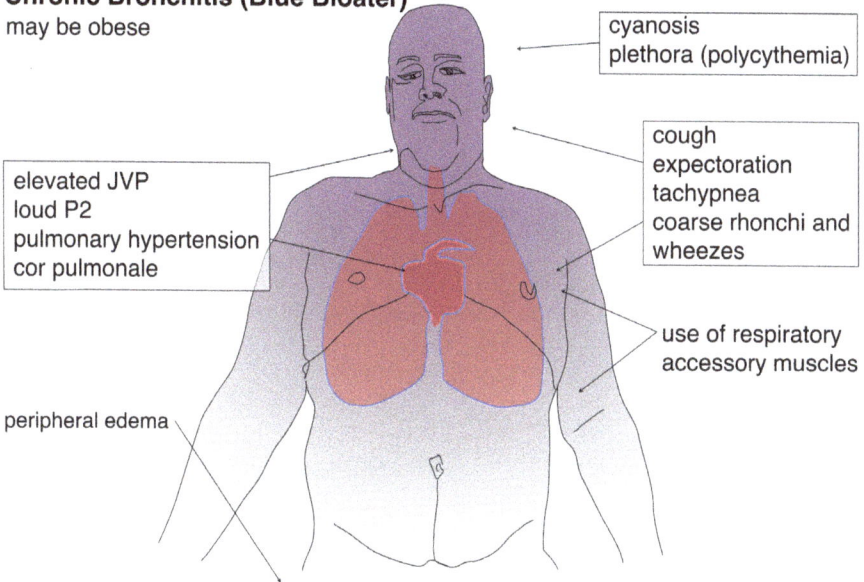

Emphysema (Pink Puffer)

may be thin

little or no cough

muscle wasting

distant heart sounds

retraction of lower
intercostal areas
(Hoover sign)

pursed lips during
expiration

hyperventilation
hyperinflated barrel chest
hyperresonant
diminished breath sounds
prolonged expiration
expiratory wheezing
coarse inspiratory crackles

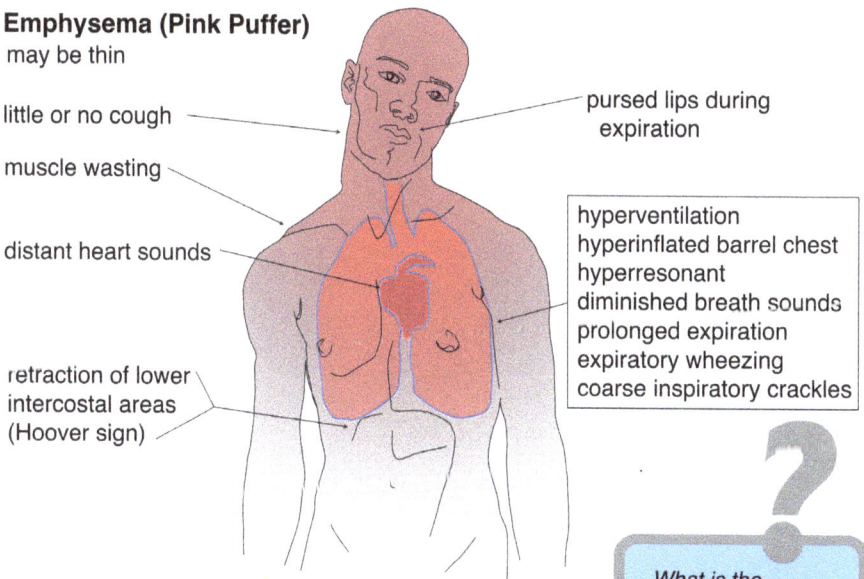

*What is the
tripod position?*

Cystic Fibrosis

Malnutrition

- vitamin deficiencies
- dry skin
- cheilosis
- nutritional or cardiac edema

Nasal

- nasal polyps
- sinusitis

Cardiac

- pulmonary hypertension
  - loud P2
  - right ventricular hypertrophy
- cor pulmonale

Pulmonary

- cyanosis
- cough
- tachypnea
- increased anteroposterior (AP) diameter
- intercostal indrawing
- hyperresonance
- wheezes, crackles
- pneumonia
- pneumothorax

Abdominal

- distension
- hepatosplenomegaly
- biliary cirrhosis
- portal hypertension
- distal intestinal obstruction
- pain, pancreatitis

Anorectal

- rectal prolapse

Rheumatologic

- hypertrophic pulmonary osteoarthropathy
- arthritis
- finger clubbing
- kyphosis, scoliosis

Cystic Fibrosis

malnutrition
- vitamin deficiencies
- dry skin
- cheilosis

nasal polyps
sinusitis

kyphosis, scoliosis

pulmonary
- cyanosis
- cough
- tachypnea
- increased AP diameter
- intercostal indrawing
- hyperresonant
- wheezes, crackles
- pneumonia
- pneumothorax

cardiac
- pulmonary hypertension
  - loud P2
  - right ventricular hypertrophy
- cor pulmonale

abdominal
- distension
- hepatosplenomegaly
- biliary cirrhosis
- portal hypertension
- pain, pancreatitis
- distal intestinal obstruction

rectal prolapse

hypertrophic
pulmonary
osteoarthropathy

finger clubbing

arthritis

nutritional or
cardiac edema

What is the sweat test?

General

- obese or overweight
- increased neck circumference (males 17", females 15")

Oropharyngeal

- narrow airway walls
- large tongue
- large tongue relative to pharynx
- high, arched palate
- enlarged tonsils ("kissing tonsils")

Dental

- retrognathia (overbite)
- marked overjet (buck teeth)

Cardiac

- arrythmias – bradyarrhythmia, ventricular extrasystoles, atrial fibrillation
- congestive heart failure
- ischemic heart disease
- myocardial infarction

Arterial

- hypertension
- atherosclerosis

Pulmonary

- pulmonary hypertension

Neurologic

- strokes
- cognitive impairment

Obstructive Sleep Apnea

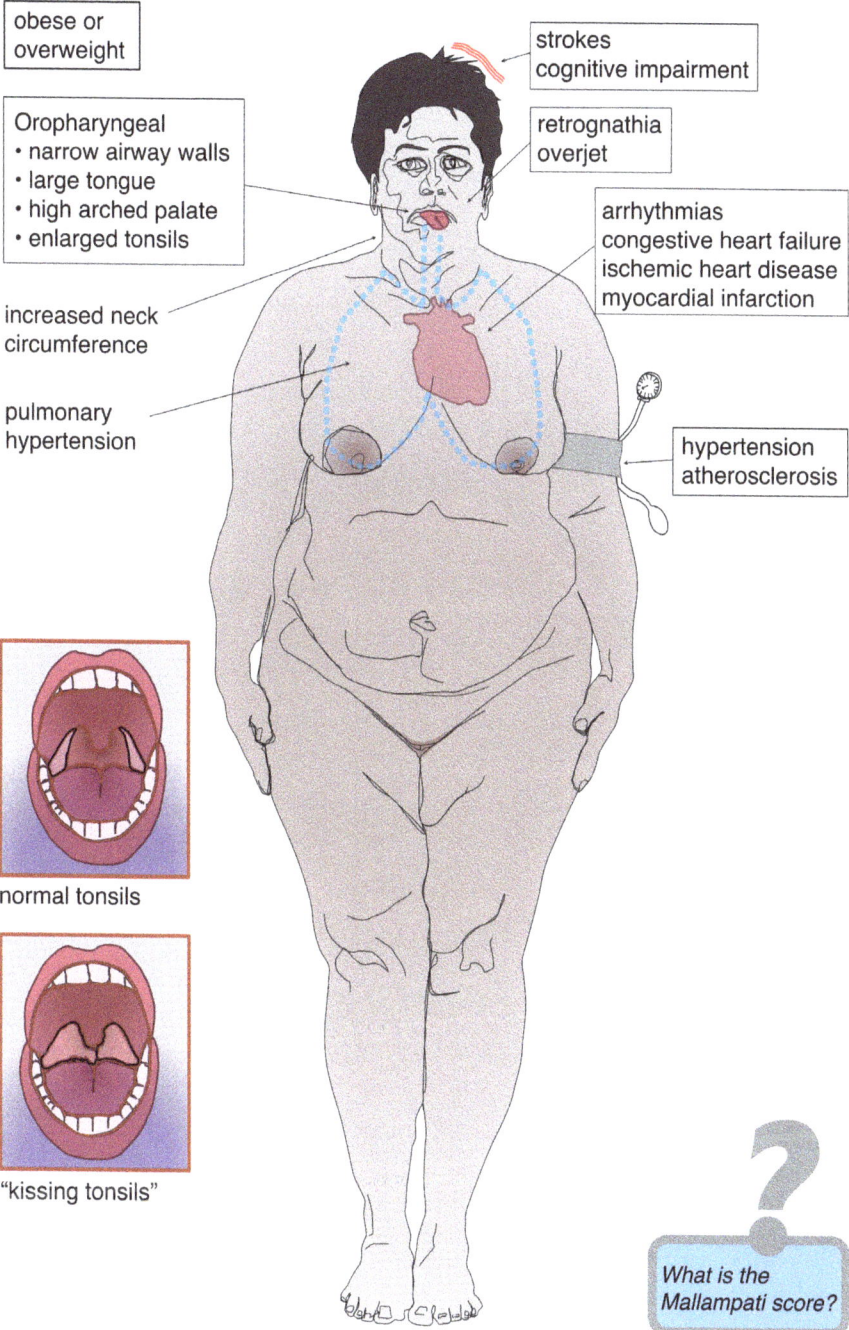

obese or overweight

strokes
cognitive impairment

Oropharyngeal
• narrow airway walls
• large tongue
• high arched palate
• enlarged tonsils

retrognathia
overjet

arrhythmias
congestive heart failure
ischemic heart disease
myocardial infarction

increased neck
circumference

pulmonary
hypertension

hypertension
atherosclerosis

normal tonsils

"kissing tonsils"

What is the
Mallampati score?

Paraneoplastic Signs of Lung Cancer

Integumentary

- acanthosis palmaris (tripe palms)
- acanthosis nigricans
- leukocytoclastic vasculitis
- thrombophlebitis migrans (Trousseau syndrome)

Endocrine

- SIADH (syndrome of inappropriate antidiuretic hormone)
- drowsiness, confusion
- ectopic ACTH (adrenocorticotropin hormone) secretion
  - muscle wasting
  - generalized hyperpigmentation
- parathyroid hormone–related protein (PTHrP) secretion
  - confusion
  - lethargy
  - thirst, increased urination
- gynecomastia

Rheumatologic

- dermatomyositis
- hypertrophic osteoarthropathy
  - finger clubbing
  - thickened ends of long bones, with pain

Neurologic

- sensorimotor polyneuropathy
- cerebellar degeneration, bilateral
  - ataxia
  - dysarthria
  - diplopia
  - nystagmus
- Lambert-Eaton myasthenia syndrome
  - muscle weakness
- autonomic neuropathies
  - intestinal pseudo-obstruction

Paraneoplastic Signs of Lung Cancer

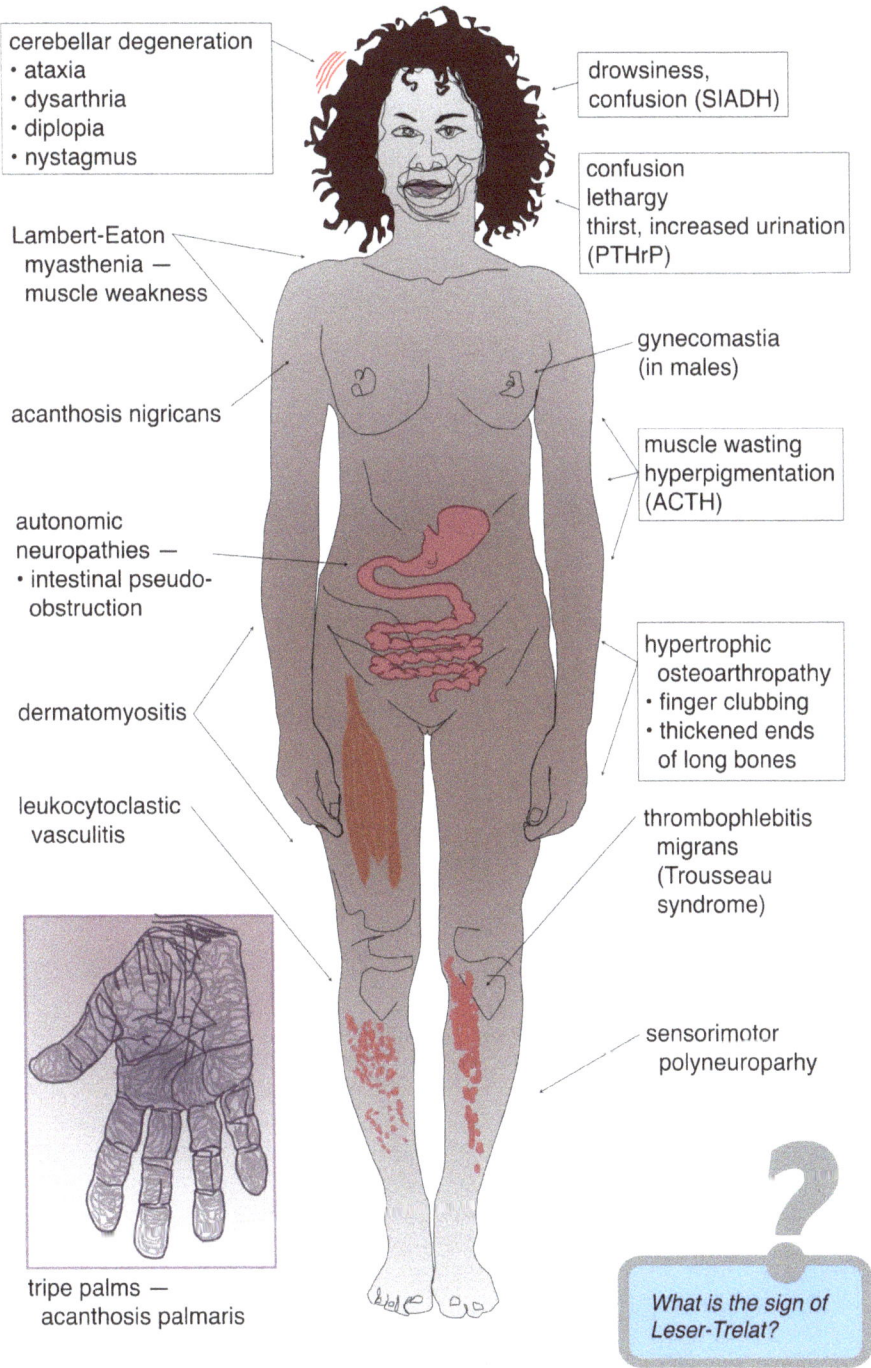

cerebellar degeneration
• ataxia
• dysarthria
• diplopia
• nystagmus

drowsiness,
confusion (SIADH)

confusion
lethargy
thirst, increased urination
(PTHrP)

Lambert-Eaton
myasthenia —
muscle weakness

gynecomastia
(in males)

acanthosis nigricans

muscle wasting
hyperpigmentation
(ACTH)

autonomic
neuropathies —
• intestinal pseudo-
  obstruction

hypertrophic
osteoarthropathy
• finger clubbing
• thickened ends
  of long bones

dermatomyositis

leukocytoclastic
vasculitis

thrombophlebitis
migrans
(Trousseau
syndrome)

sensorimotor
polyneuroparhy

tripe palms —
acanthosis palmaris

What is the sign of
Leser-Trelat?

Ocular

- uveitis and episcleritis
- vitreous opacities
- optic disc nodules
- choroidal nodules

Otorhinolaryngologic

- otitis media
- hearing loss
- anosmia
- nasal mucosal inflammation, crusting
- xerostomia

Exocrine

- bilateral parotid gland enlargement

Lymphatic

- lymphadenopathy – cervical, epitrochlear, inguinal

Integumentary

- erythema nodosum
- plaques, papules
- subcutaneous nodules
- lupus pernio: violaceous papules, plaques around nose, cheeks, ears
- inflammation, induration around scars and tattoos

Cardiac

- heart block
- palpitations, tachyarrhythmias

Abdominal

- splenomegaly

Rheumatologic

- acute oligoarthritis
- polyarthritis

Neurologic

- cranial nerve palsies
- bilateral facial nerve palsy

Löfgren syndrome: erythema nodosum, bilateral hilar adenopathy, polyarthralgia

---

Heerfordt syndrome (uveoparotid fever): parotid gland enlargement, fever, facial palsy, anterior uveitis

---

Sarcoidosis
Extrapulmonary Signs

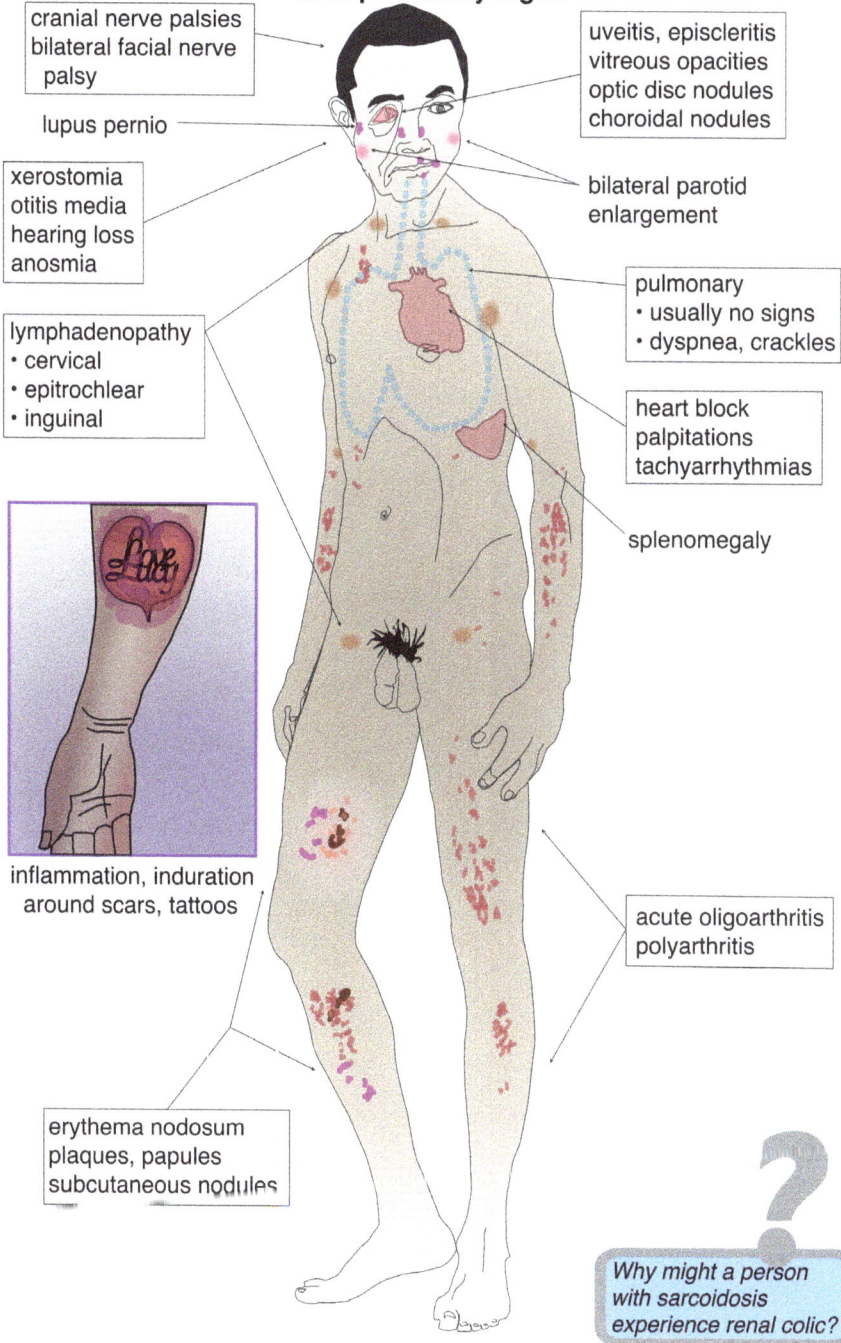

cranial nerve palsies
bilateral facial nerve
  palsy

lupus pernio

xerostomia
otitis media
hearing loss
anosmia

lymphadenopathy
• cervical
• epitrochlear
• inguinal

uveitis, episcleritis
vitreous opacities
optic disc nodules
choroidal nodules

bilateral parotid
enlargement

pulmonary
• usually no signs
• dyspnea, crackles

heart block
palpitations
tachyarrhythmias

splenomegaly

inflammation, induration
around scars, tattoos

acute oligoarthritis
polyarthritis

erythema nodosum
plaques, papules
subcutaneous nodules

*Why might a person
with sarcoidosis
experience renal colic?*

RHEUMATOLOGY

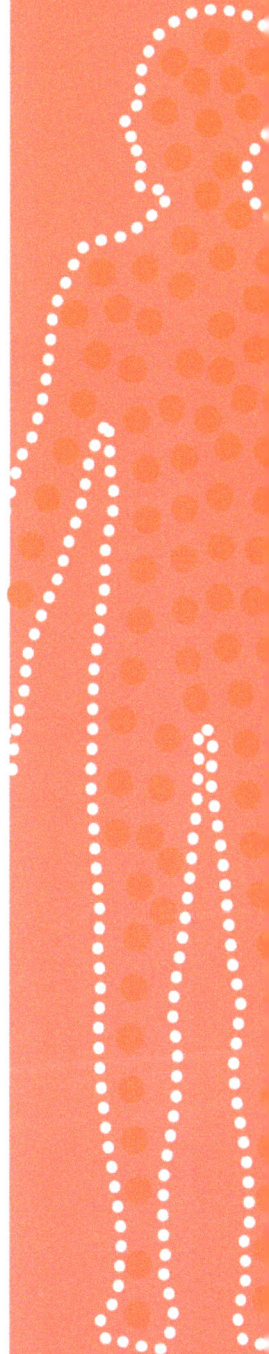

ARTICULAR SIGNS

Spinal

- stiff spine with limited mobility
- stooped posture
- cervical spine forward flexion ("chin on chest")
- dorsal kyphosis, upper thoracic spine
- loss of lumbar lordosis, flattening of lumbar spine
- spine fractures
- tender spine and sacroiliac (SI) joints

Synovial

- synovitis
  - shoulders
  - hips
  - knees
  - temporomandibular (TM) joints

Enthesial

- enthesitis,* causing pain and tenderness
  - heels
  - Achilles tendons
  - tibial tuberosities
  - iliac crests
  - supra- and infrapatellar tendons
  - costosternal, costovertebral joints
  - sternomanubrial joints

*Enthesitis: inflammation of the enthesis, i.e., the insertion site where tendons and ligaments attach to bone

EXTRAARTICULAR SIGNS

Ocular

- anterior uveitis (painful, red eye)

Cardiac

- aortitis, aortic regurgitation
- conduction disturbance, possibly complete heart block

Pulmonary

- restricted chest expansion, <5 cm

Abdominal

- pain

Neurologic

- cervical myelopathy (C1–C2 subluxation)
- cauda equina syndrome

Ankylosing Spondylitis

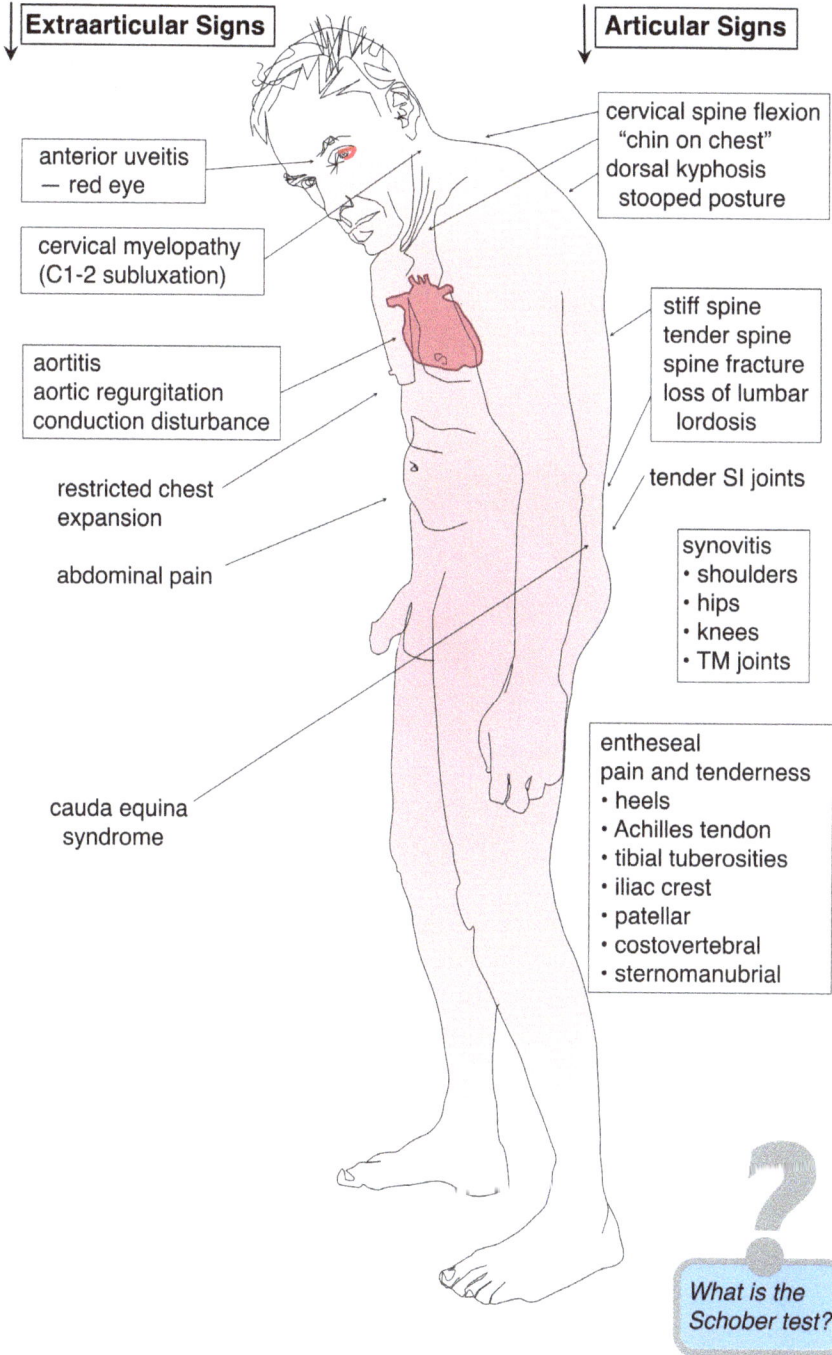

anterior uveitis
— red eye

cervical myelopathy
(C1-2 subluxation)

aortitis
aortic regurgitation
conduction disturbance

restricted chest
expansion

abdominal pain

cauda equina
syndrome

cervical spine flexion
"chin on chest"
dorsal kyphosis
stooped posture

stiff spine
tender spine
spine fracture
loss of lumbar
lordosis

tender SI joints

synovitis
• shoulders
• hips
• knees
• TM joints

entheseal
pain and tenderness
• heels
• Achilles tendon
• tibial tuberosities
• iliac crest
• patellar
• costovertebral
• sternomanubrial

What is the Schober test?

Granulomatosis with Polyangiitis (GPA) (Wegener Granulomatosis)

Ocular
- conjunctivitis
- uveitis
- episcleritis
- proptosis (orbital pseudotumor)
- retinal vasculitis

Nasal
- epistaxis
- sinusitis
- saddle nose deformity

Auditory
- hearing loss

Oral
- strawberry gingival hyperplasia

Integumentary
- digital infarcts
- palpable purpura
- livedo reticularis
- subungual splinter hemorrhages
- vasculitis – varied, ulcers, nodules, infarcts

Cardiac
- pericardial rub
- myocardial infarction

Pulmonary
- cough, hoarseness
- subglottic stridor
- hemoptysis
- pleural effusion
- adventitious sounds – cavitation, atelectasis

Abdominal
- pain and tenderness (splanchnic vasculitis)

Renal
- edema (renal vasculitis)

Rheumatologic
- arthritis
- polyarthritis

Neurologic
- mononeuritis multiplex
- sensorimotor polyneuropathy
- cranial nerve palsies

Granulomatosis with Polyangiitis (GPA)
(Wegener Granulomatosis)

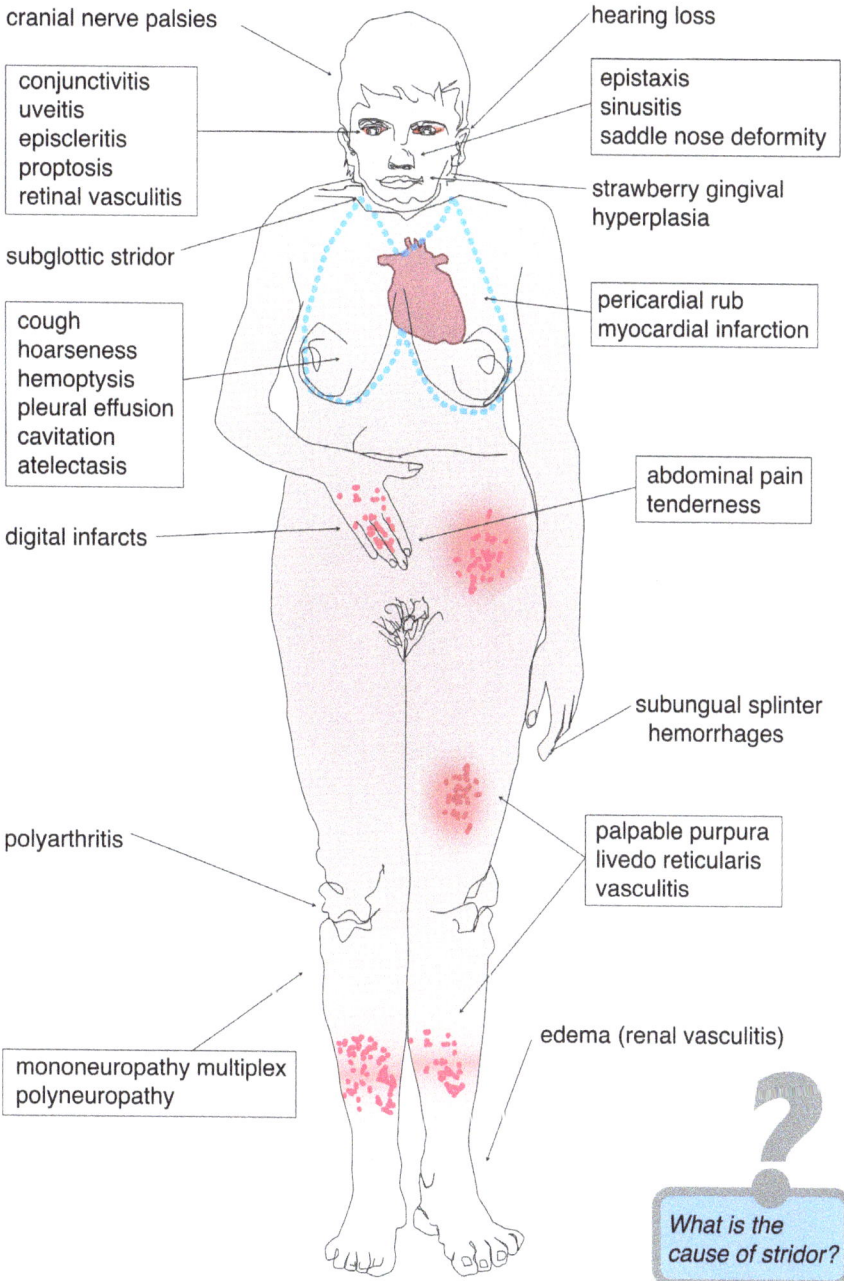

cranial nerve palsies

hearing loss

conjunctivitis
uveitis
episcleritis
proptosis
retinal vasculitis

epistaxis
sinusitis
saddle nose deformity

strawberry gingival
hyperplasia

subglottic stridor

pericardial rub
myocardial infarction

cough
hoarseness
hemoptysis
pleural effusion
cavitation
atelectasis

abdominal pain
tenderness

digital infarcts

subungual splinter
hemorrhages

polyarthritis

palpable purpura
livedo reticularis
vasculitis

edema (renal vasculitis)

mononeuropathy multiplex
polyneuropathy

What is the cause of stridor?

Rheumatoid Arthritis (RA)

ARTICULAR SIGNS*

Symmetrical Joints

- morning stiffness
- tenderness and limitation of movement
- deformities
- tenosynovitis

Hands and Wrists

- carpal tunnel syndrome
- ulnar deviation of phalanges
- radial deviation of metacarpals
- proximal interphalangeal (PIP) joint swelling
- boutonniere (buttonhole) and swan neck finger deformities

Feet

- pes planus ("flat feet")
- hammer toes
- hallux valgus
- callouses

Knees

- limitation of movement
- flexion deformity
- Baker cyst

Cervical Spine

- cervical spine arthritis, stiff neck
- C1–C2 subluxation

*RA can affect any synovial joint, with some joints more classically involved.

EXTRAARTICULAR SIGNS

Ocular

- episcleritis
- keratitis
- keratoconjunctivitis sicca

Cutaneous

- nodules
  - extensor surfaces, especially elbows
  - vasculitis, digital arteritis
  - cutaneous vasculitis
  - pyoderma gangrenosum

Cardiac

- pericarditis
- myocarditis
- coronary arteritis
- conduction defects
- aortitis

Pulmonary

- pleural effusion
- lung crackles (interstitial lung disease)

Abdominal

- splenomegaly (in Felty syndrome)

Neurologic

- peripheral neuropathies
- mononeuritis multiplex
- compression neuropathies
- cervical cord compression

Rheumatoid Arthritis (RA)

↓ Articular Signs

symmetrical arthritis
of any synovial joint
morning stiffness

C1-C2 arthritis
subluxation

carpal tunnel syndrome
radial deviation of
 metacarpals
ulnar deviation of
 phalanges
PIP joint swelling
boutonniere and
 swan neck fingers

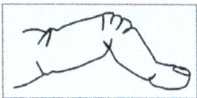

limitation of
 movement
flexion deformity
knee arthritis
synovitis
Baker cyst

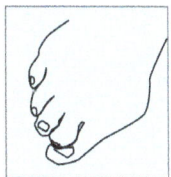

hammer toes

hammer toes
pes planus
hallux valgus
callouses

↓ Extraarticular Signs

episcleritis
keratitis
keratoconjunctivitis sicca

cervical cord compression

pericarditis
myocarditis
coronary arteritis
conduction defects
aortitis

pleural effusion
lung crackles

nodules
 (extensor surfaces)

splenomegaly

compression
 neuropathies

digital arteritis
cutaneous vasculitis
pyoderma gangrenosum

peripheral neuropathy
mononeuritis multiplex

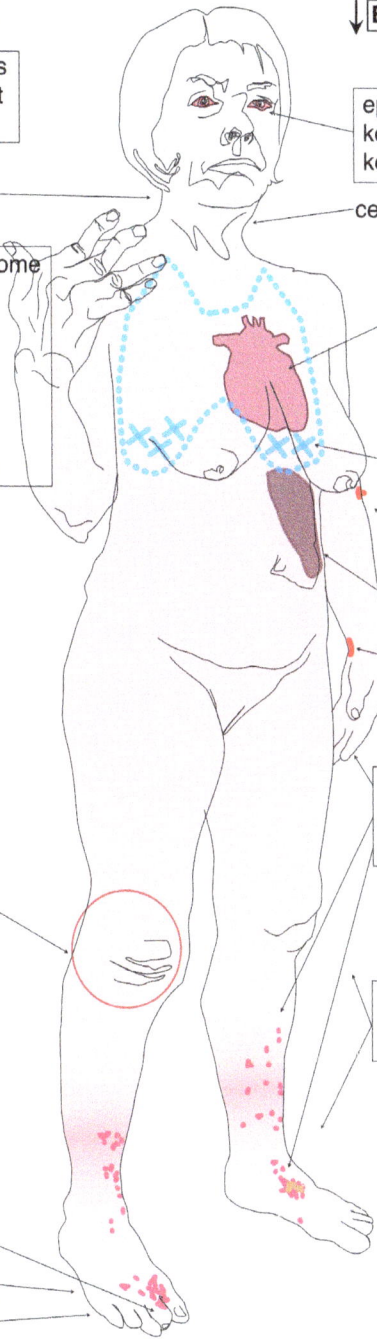

What is Felty
syndrome?

Scleroderma

Ocular
- keratoconjunctivitis sicca

Oral
- microstoma, decreased oral aperture
- xerostomia (dry mouth)

Integumentary
- thin, dry skin
- tight, decreased skin folds
- loss of body hair
- hyper- and hypopigmentation ("salt and pepper" appearance)
- telangiectasia – face, hands, anterior chest
- calcinosis – fingertips, extensor forearms, prepatellar area
- sclerodactyly
- infarction, dry gangrene of fingers and toes
- Raynaud phenomenon

Cardiac
- conduction disturbances, arrhythmias
- cardiomyopathy
- increased P2
- pericardial effusion

Arterial
- accelerated hypertension

Pulmonary
- fine, dry crackles
- flash pulmonary edema

Abdominal
- distended abdomen (intestinal pseudo-obstruction)

Rheumatologic
- myositis
- arthritis
- flexion contractures
- palpable tendon friction rub

Neurologic
- cranial neuropathies
- peripheral neuropathy
- carpal tunnel syndrome

Scleroderma

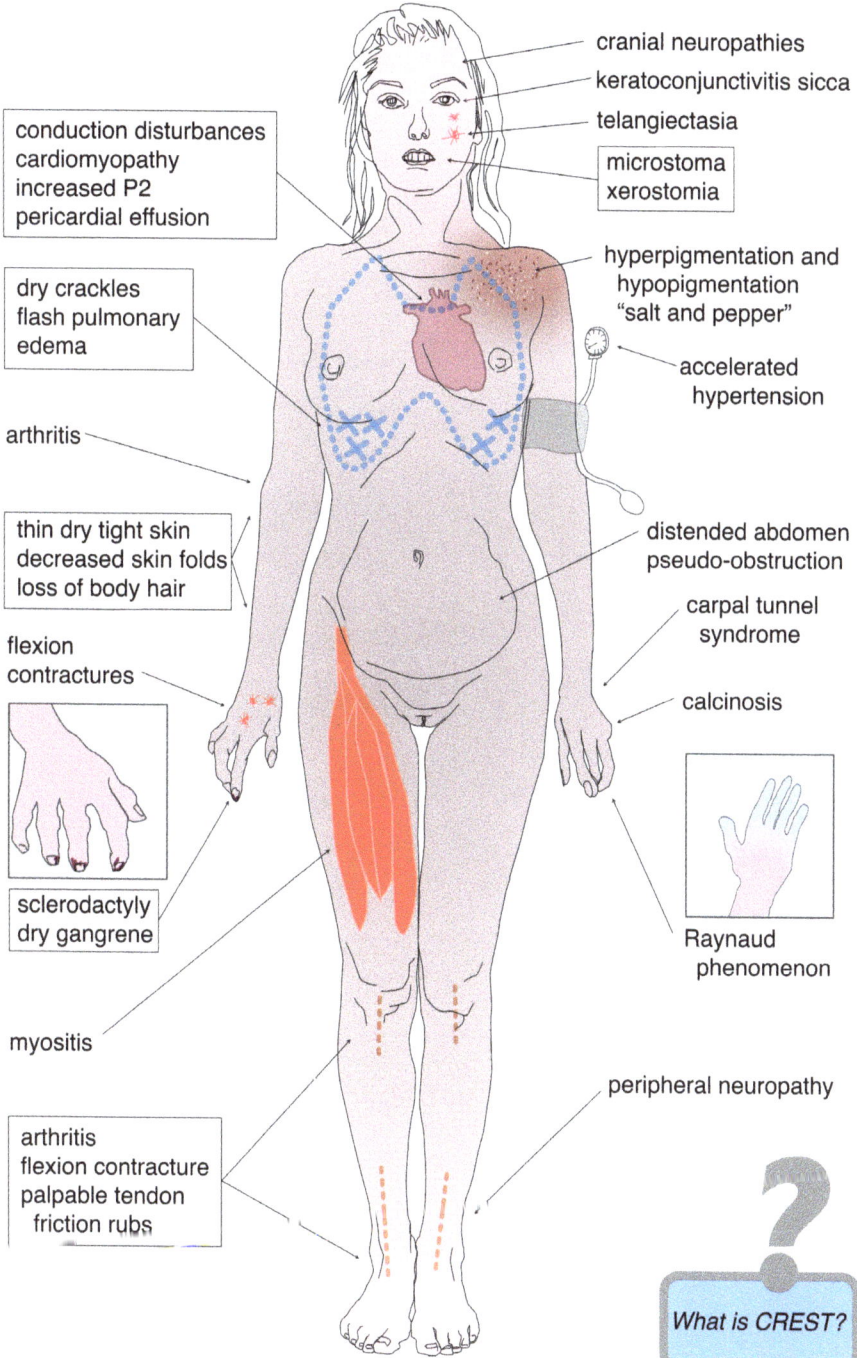

cranial neuropathies

keratoconjunctivitis sicca

telangiectasia

microstoma
xerostomia

conduction disturbances
cardiomyopathy
increased P2
pericardial effusion

hyperpigmentation and
hypopigmentation
"salt and pepper"

accelerated
hypertension

dry crackles
flash pulmonary
edema

arthritis

thin dry tight skin
decreased skin folds
loss of body hair

distended abdomen
pseudo-obstruction

carpal tunnel
syndrome

calcinosis

flexion
contractures

sclerodactyly
dry gangrene

Raynaud
phenomenon

myositis

peripheral neuropathy

arthritis
flexion contracture
palpable tendon
 friction rubs

What is CREST?

Sjögren Syndrome

GLANDULAR SIGNS

Ocular
- keratoconjunctivitis sicca
- keratitis
- blepharitis
- dilated conjunctival vessels (red eyes)

Nasal
- dry nose, crusting

Oral
- xerostomia (dry mouth)
- dental caries
- cheilitis
- oral candidiasis

Exocrine
- parotid gland enlargement (bilateral)
- other exocrine gland atrophy, dryness
  - nasal, upper respiratory
  - vulvar, vaginal
  - anal, rectal

EXTRAGLANDULAR SIGNS

Lymphatic
- lymphadenopathy

Integumentary
- xeroderma (dry skin)
- vasculitis
- purpura
- urticaria
- annular erythema
- Raynaud phenomenon

Pulmonary
- bibasilar crackles (interstitial lung disease)

Abdominal
- splenomegaly

Rheumatologic
- myalgias
- polyarthritis

Neuropsychiatric
- neuropsychiatric problems
- peripheral neuropathy

Sjögren Syndrome

dry nose, crusting

neuropsychiatric problems

dry mouth
dental caries
cheilitis
oral candidiasis

keratoconjuntivitis sicca
keratitis
blepharitis
red eyes

bibasalar crackles

parotid gland enlargement

lymphadenopathy

splenomegaly

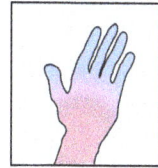

dry skin
vasculitis
purpura
urticaria
annular erythema
Raynaud
  phenomenon

Raynaud
phenomenon

vulvar and
vaginal dryness

myalgias
polyarthritis

peripheral neuropathy

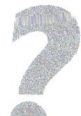

What is the
Schirmer test?

Systemic Lupus Erythematosus (SLE)

SLE is an autoimmune disease that can affect any organ in variable ways.

General

- fever
- weight loss
- anemia

Ocular

- lupus retinitis – exudates, vascular changes
- keratoconjunctivitis sicca

Oral

- mouth ulcers

Lymphatic

- lymphadenopathy

Integumentary

- malar butterfly rash
- discoid rash
- photosensitivity rashes – macular erythema
- patchy alopecia
- livedo reticularis
- telangiectasia
- Raynaud phenomenon

Cardiac

- pericarditis
- myocarditis
- cardiac murmurs, valvular disease
- endocarditis (Libman-Sacks endocarditis)

Arterial

- hypertension

Pulmonary

- lung crackles
- pleuritis
- pneumonitis
- interstitial lung disease
- pulmonary hemorrhage
- pulmonary hypertension

Abdominal

- pain – peritonitis, pancreatitis, mesenteric vasculitis
- splenomegaly

Renal

- nephrotic edema

Rheumatologic

- polyarthritis
- metacarpophalangeal (MCP), proximal interphalangeal (PIP) joint and wrist arthritis
- nonerosive hand deformities (Jaccoud arthropathy)
- myositis

Neuropsychiatric

- psychosis
- seizures
- demyelinating syndromes
- peripheral neuropathy

Systemic Lupus Erythematosis (SLE)

fever
weight loss
anemia

patchy alopecia

malar butterfly rash
discoid rash

mouth ulcers

psychosis
seizures
demyelinating syndromes

lupus retinitis
keratoconjunctivitis sicca

pericarditis
myocarditis
murmurs
Libman-Sacks
 endocarditis
hypertension

lymphadenopathy

crackles
pleuritis
pneumonitis
interstitial disease
hemorrhage
pulmonary
 hypertension

splenomegaly
abdominal pain

photosensitivity rashes
— macular erythematous

polyarthritis
• MCP & PIP joints
• wrist joints
• Jaccoud
 arthropathy

Raynaud
phenomenon

livedo reticularis

myositis

telangiectasia

peripheral neuropathy

nephrotic odema

What is shrinking
lung syndrome?

DO IT YOURSELF

Use the following pages for additional syndromes—create lists of clinical signs for each and annotate the patient figures.

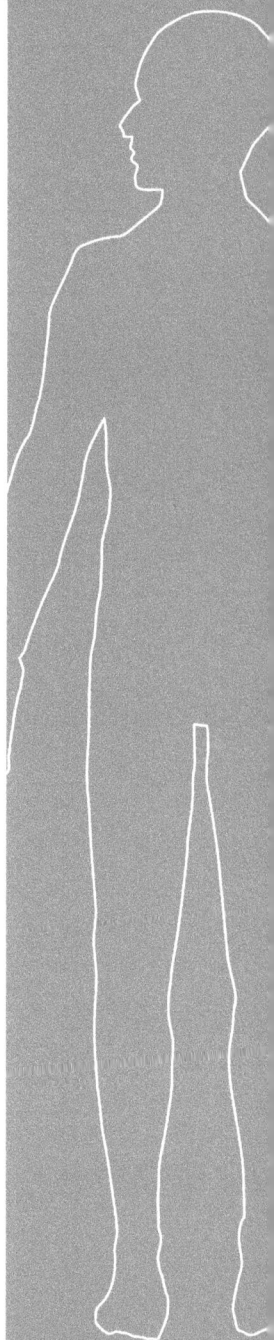

Do It Yourself

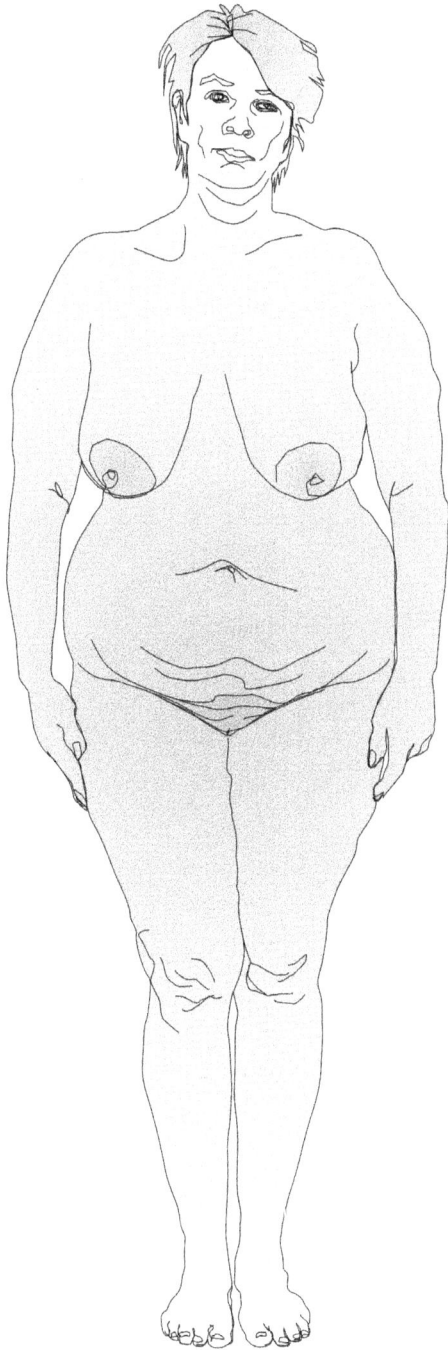

Do It Yourself

....

....

....

....

....

....

....

....

....

....

....

....

....

....

....

....

....

....

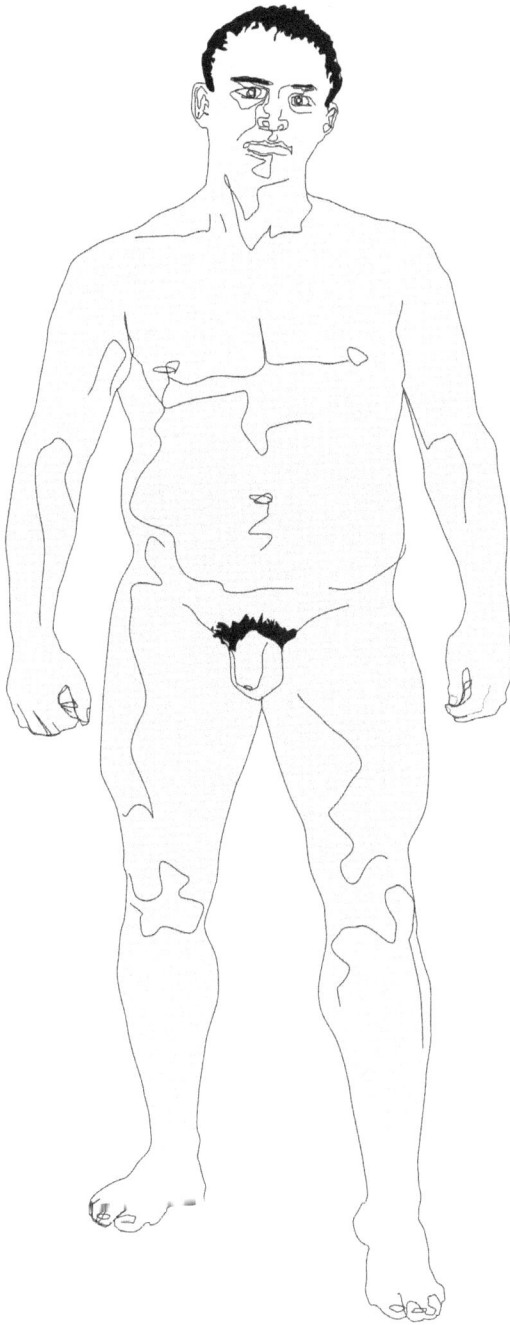

Do It Yourself

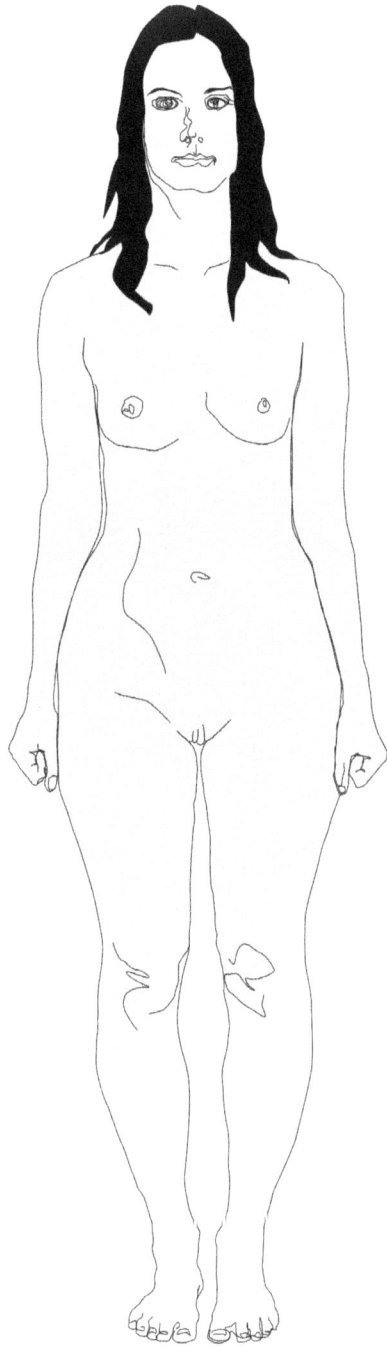

....

....

....

....

....

....

....

....

....

....

....

....

....

....

....

....

....

....

....

....

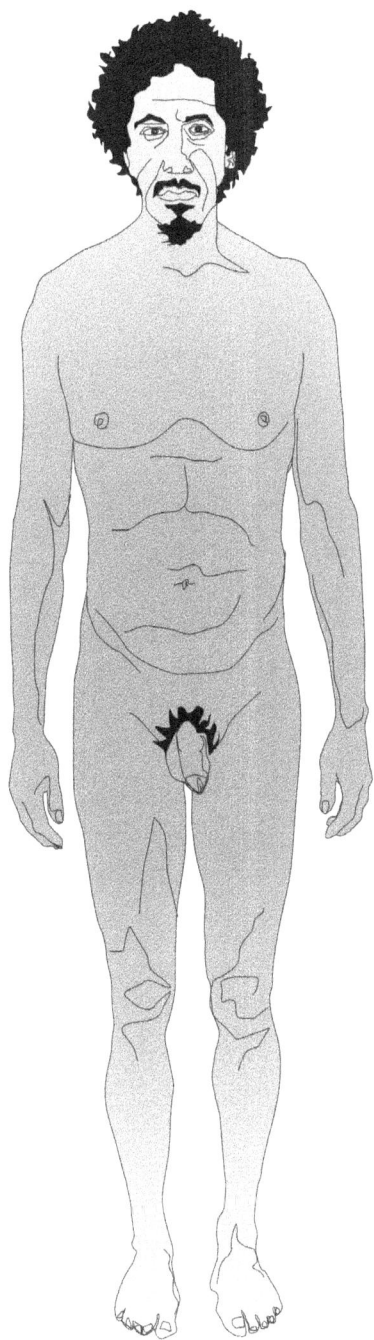

Do It Yourself

....

....

....

....

....

....

....

....

....

....

....

....

....

....

....

....

....

....

....

....

....

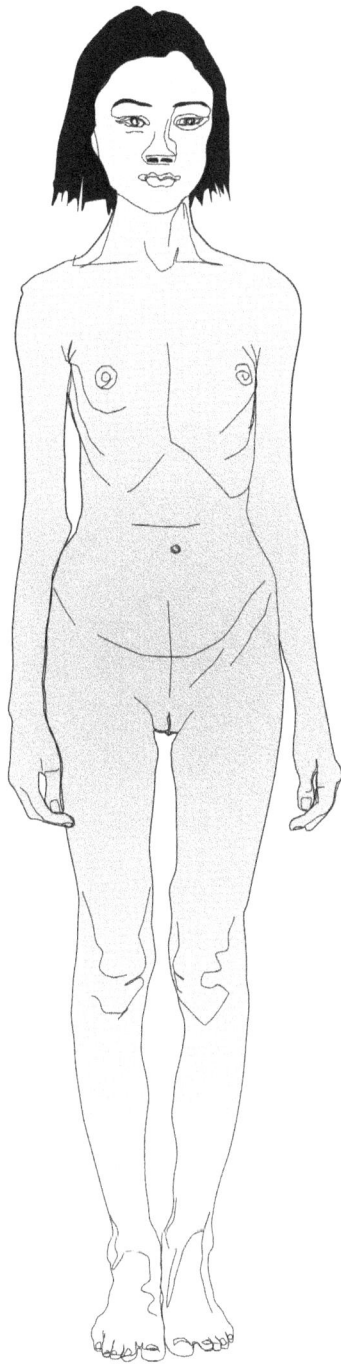

Do It Yourself

. . . .

. . . .

. . . .

. . . .

. . . .

. . . .

. . . .

. . . .

. . . .

. . . .

. . . .

. . . .

. . . .

. . . .

. . . .

. . . .

. . . .

. . . .

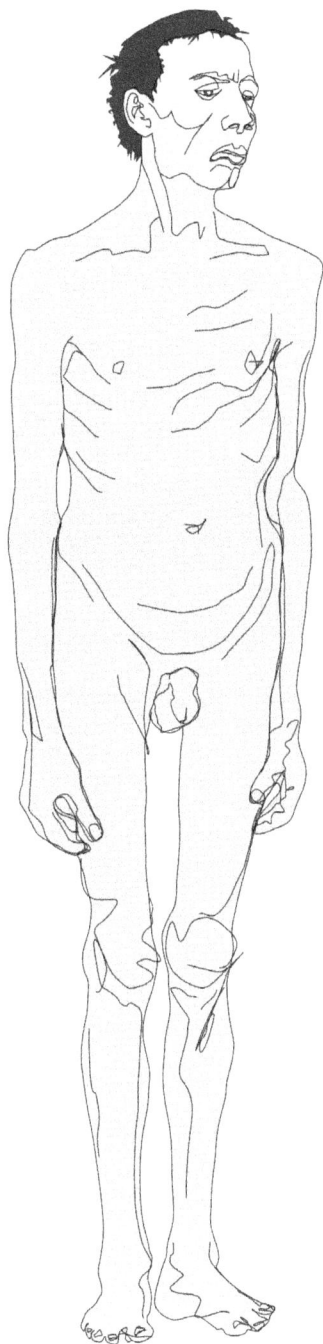

INDEX

We would like to thank the following people:

- the students, residents and colleagues, for always challenging and inspirng.
- our editor, Kelly Davis, for adding coherence to this project.
- Patty Osborne of Vancouver Desktop Publishing Centre, for her layout expertise and infinite patience.
- Lisa of Index Busters, for making things findable.
- most importantly, and with much affection, our wives, Lorna, and Cindy, for their helpful comments and unfailing support.

Contributors

Clifford Chan-Yan, MBChB, FRCPC

Clifford Chan-Yan is a clinical professor emeritus at the University of British Columbia, Canada. He received his medical degree from the University of Cape Town and a specialty in internal medicine from the College of Physicians of South Africa and the Royal College of Physicians of Canada. He is a former examiner for the Royal College's final clinical examinations. As a clinical instructor with an interest in physical examination, he endeavors to teach this practical skill to others.

Eldon Underhill

Eldon Underhill is a visual artist with more than thirty-five years of experience in graphic art, design, and illustration. During his twenty-year graphic design career at St. Paul's Hospital in Vancouver, Canada, he worked with physicians and other health professionals to develop a wide variety of materials related to both patient education and professional communication. He graduated from the former Vancouver School of Art (now Emily Carr University of Art and Design) in 1977. He maintains both a graphic design and fine art (painting and photography) practice at his home in Halfmoon Bay, Canada.

www.ingramcontent.com/pod-product-compliance
Lightning Source LLC
Chambersburg PA
CBHW040925210326
41597CB00030B/5179